TESTED TECHNIQUES TO GETTING RID OF DIABETES NATUALLY

THE AMAZING POWER OF NATURE

ABIK ALEXANDER

DEDICATION

This book is dedicated to my lovely wife, Mrs. Alexander Yem.

CONTENTS

ACKNOWLEDGMENTS

Tested Techniques to Getting Rid of Diabetes Naturally, is the result of the efforts of many people, all of whom deserve my sincere gratitude. Above all else, I'm obliged to the devoted scientists and medical services experts whose resolute endeavors have prepared for regular diabetes the executives. I also want to express my gratitude to the brave people who bravely shared their personal struggles and triumphs, inspiring and reassuring others on this journey. In conclusion, I'm grateful to my family, companions, and the distributing group for their faithful help and consolation all through this groundbreaking undertaking.

Abik Alexander

CHAPTER ONE

INTRODUCTION TO DIABETES

Millions of people around the world suffer from **diabetes,** a chronic metabolic condition. It is described by raised glucose levels because of either deficient insulin creation or the body's powerlessness to use insulin successfully. The pancreas produces insulin, a hormone that regulates blood sugar levels and makes it easier for glucose to enter cells for energy production.

Diabetes is primarily divided into three categories: gestational diabetes, type 1 diabetes, and type 2 diabetes. The immune system mistakenly attacks and destroys the insulin-producing cells in the pancreas, resulting in type 1 diabetes. As a result, there is no insulin at all, requiring insulin injections or the use of an insulin pump for the rest of one's life. On the other hand, type 2 diabetes typically occurs later in life and is characterized by insulin resistance, in which the body becomes less responsive to insulin's effects. Although gestational diabetes usually goes away after a child is born, it can make it more likely that a person will develop type 2 diabetes in later life.

The pervasiveness of diabetes has been consistently ascending throughout the course of recent many years, basically determined by changes in way of life and an expansion in stoutness rates. Uncontrolled diabetes can prompt different entanglements, including coronary illness, stroke, kidney harm, nerve harm, and vision issues. As a result, effective diabetes management is essential for avoiding these complications and maintaining a high quality of life.

Diabetes management requires a comprehensive strategy that

incorporates diet, exercise, stress management, medication, and other lifestyle choices. Diabetes patients often need to take medication, but there are also a number of natural methods that can be used to control blood sugar levels and improve overall health.

Changing one's lifestyle is an essential part of natural diabetes management. Taking on a sound way of life that incorporates a fair eating routine, customary activity, and stress the executives methods can essentially affect diabetes control. Blood sugar levels can be controlled with a well-planned meal plan that emphasizes whole foods that are high in fiber and low in processed sugars and carbohydrates. Improved insulin sensitivity and weight loss can both be aided by physical activity, which is especially helpful for people with type 2 diabetes.

Certain natural foods and herbs have been found to have blood sugar-lowering properties in addition to lifestyle changes. For instance, food varieties like verdant green vegetables, berries, nuts, and seeds are known to be helpful for diabetes the board. Cinnamon, fenugreek, and turmeric, among other herbs and spices, have also demonstrated the capacity to lower blood sugar levels. However, it is essential to keep in mind that these natural remedies should not be used in place of prescription medications; rather, they should be used in conjunction with medical advice.

Other essential methods for naturally managing diabetes include mindful eating and portion control. Diabetes patients can maintain more stable blood sugar levels and avoid overeating by paying attention to hunger and fullness cues. When it comes to carbohydrate-rich foods, portion control is especially important because they directly affect blood sugar levels. People can better control their glycemic control and blood sugar levels by monitoring and controlling portion sizes.

Stress the board and quality rest likewise assume a pivotal part in diabetes the executives. Stress reduction strategies like deep breathing exercises, hobbies, and meditation can be helpful because chronic stress can raise blood sugar levels. Lack of sleep can have an impact on insulin sensitivity and blood sugar regulation, so getting enough quality sleep is just as important.

For diabetes management to be successful, it is necessary to monitor blood sugar levels on a regular basis in addition to keeping track of food, exercise, and medication. Individuals can identify patterns, make necessary adjustments, and celebrate milestones in their diabetes control journey by keeping track of these factors. Diabetes tracking and management can be made easier with the help of technology like Smartphone applications and glucose monitoring devices.

Understanding the fundamentals of diabetes is important because diabetes is a chronic metabolic disorder that affects millions of people around the world. It is characterized by high blood sugar levels, or hyperglycemia, which can be caused by the body not making enough insulin or not using insulin properly. The pancreas produces insulin, a hormone that regulates blood sugar levels and makes it easier for glucose to enter cells for energy production.

Diabetes is primarily divided into three categories: type 1 diabetes, type 2 diabetes, and gestational diabetes.

Type 1 Diabetes:

Type 1 diabetes for the most part grows from the get-go throughout everyday life, frequently during youth or immaturity. It occurs when the pancreas' insulin-producing cells are mistakenly attacked and destroyed by the immune system, resulting in low or no insulin production. To control their blood sugar levels, people with type 1 diabetes must take insulin injections or use an insulin pump for the rest of their lives. Although the exact cause of type 1 diabetes is still unknown, a combination of genetic and environmental factors is thought to be the cause.

Diabetes de type 2:

The majority of cases of diabetes are of type 2, the most prevalent form. It ordinarily grows sometime down the road, in spite of the fact that it is progressively being analyzed in more youthful people because of increasing heftiness rates. In type 2 diabetes, the pancreas fails to produce enough insulin to meet the body's needs, or the body becomes resistant to the effects of insulin. This outcomes in raised glucose levels. Obesity, a sedentary lifestyle, a poor diet, a diabetes history in the family, and certain ethnic backgrounds are all risk factors for type 2 diabetes. In contrast to type 1 diabetes, type 2 diabetes can frequently be managed through lifestyle changes like eating a healthy diet, getting more exercise, and losing weight. Now and again, oral meds or insulin may likewise be recommended.

Diabetes at Birth:

Gestational diabetes usually goes away after a child is born. It usually happens during pregnancy. High blood sugar levels during pregnancy in women who did not have diabetes before becoming pregnant are characteristic of this condition. The chemicals created during pregnancy can obstruct the body's insulin activity, prompting insulin opposition. Gestational diabetes can raise the risk of complications during pregnancy and delivery, as well as the likelihood that both the mother and the child will develop type 2 diabetes in later life. Glucose checking, dietary changes, and some of the time prescription are important to oversee gestational diabetes.

Uncontrolled diabetes can have serious wellbeing results. Over time, high blood sugar levels can cause damage to a number of the body's organs and systems, which can lead to problems like heart disease, stroke, kidney disease, nerve damage (neuropathy), eye problems (retinopathy), and foot problems. As a result, diabetes patients need to be able to effectively manage their condition.

A multifaceted approach to diabetes management includes regular blood sugar monitoring, adopting a healthy lifestyle, taking medication (if necessary), and continuing education and support. People can monitor their blood sugar levels with blood sugar monitoring, which enables them to adjust their diet, exercise, and medication as necessary to maintain stable blood sugar control. A healthy diet, regular exercise, managing one's weight, reducing stress, and getting enough sleep are all important aspects of a diabetes management lifestyle. When lifestyle changes alone are insufficient, medication, such as insulin or oral medications, may be prescribed to assist in controlling blood sugar levels.

All in all, diabetes is an ongoing metabolic problem described by raised glucose levels. Understanding the various types of diabetes, including type 1, type 2, and gestational diabetes, is essential because each requires its own unique management strategies. By observing glucose levels, taking on a sound way of life, and heeding clinical guidance, people with diabetes can really deal with their condition and diminish the gamble of complexities, empowering them to carry on with a solid and satisfying life.

Types of diabetes and their causes Diabetes is a metabolic disorder that occurs over time and is characterized by high blood sugar levels. Diabetes comes in many different forms, each with its own causes and characteristics. Understanding the various kinds can assist people with dealing with their condition successfully and arrive at informed conclusions about their treatment choices. Type 1 diabetes, type 2 diabetes, and gestational diabetes are the most common types of diabetes.

TYPE 1 DIABETES:

Type 1 diabetes, also known as juvenile-onset diabetes or insulin-dependent diabetes, typically appears in childhood or adolescence. The immune system mistakenly attacks and destroys the insulin-producing cells in the pancreas in this autoimmune disease. Thus, the pancreas creates next to zero insulin, prompting a lack of this critical chemical. Although the exact cause of type 1 diabetes is unknown, it is thought to involve both genetic and environmental factors. In people with a genetic predisposition to the disease, certain dietary factors and viral infections may trigger the autoimmune response, according to some research. Type 1 diabetes cannot be prevented and requires insulin therapy for life to control blood sugar.

TYPE 2 DIABETES:

Type 2 diabetes is the most widely recognized type of diabetes, representing most of cases around the world. It ordinarily creates in adulthood, in spite of the fact that it is progressively being analyzed in kids and young people because of increasing stoutness rates. In type 2 diabetes, the body becomes impervious with the impacts of insulin, or the pancreas neglects to deliver sufficient insulin to fulfill the body's needs. As a result, blood sugar levels rise. Type 2 diabetes is caused by a combination of genetics, obesity, a sedentary lifestyle, a poor diet, and aging. The risk of developing type 2 diabetes is also increased by ethnicity (such as African, Hispanic, or Asian), family history of diabetes, and gestational diabetes. Type 2 diabetes, in contrast to type 1 diabetes, can frequently be managed through changes to one's lifestyle, such as losing weight, engaging in regular physical activity, and altering one's diet. When insulin sensitivity needs to be increased or insulin production stimulated, oral anti-diabetic medications may be prescribed.

DIABETES AT BIRTH:

Gestational diabetes typically manifests itself between the 24th and 28th weeks of pregnancy. It is brought on by hormonal changes that result in insulin resistance, and it only affects a small percentage of pregnant women. During pregnancy, the placenta produces chemicals that can impede the body's insulin activity, bringing about raised glucose levels. Even though gestational diabetes usually goes away after birth, it can cause problems for both the mother and the baby. Women who have diabetes during pregnancy are more likely to develop type 2 diabetes in later life. Being overweight or obese, having a family history of diabetes, being older than 25, and having certain ethnic backgrounds (such as African, Hispanic, or Asian descent) are all risk factors for gestational diabetes. In order to control gestational diabetes and ensure a healthy pregnancy, blood sugar monitoring, dietary modifications, and occasionally medication are required.

It is essential to keep in mind that there are additional, less prevalent forms of diabetes, such as drug-induced diabetes, monogenic diabetes (caused by a single gene mutation), and monogenic diabetes (caused by a single gene mutation). These varieties may necessitate specialized management strategies due to specific underlying causes.

In conclusion, there are many different kinds of diabetes, each of which has its own causes and characteristics. The pancreas destroys insulin-producing cells, resulting in type 1 diabetes, an autoimmune condition. Type 2 diabetes is essentially connected with insulin obstruction and insufficient insulin creation, frequently affected by hereditary and way of life factors. Gestational diabetes happens during pregnancy because of hormonal changes that lead to insulin opposition. For effective management and prevention, it is essential to comprehend the causes of these diabetes types as well as their distinct characteristics.

Diabetes is a chronic condition that must be managed throughout one's life to avoid complications and preserve a high quality of life. While prescription is many times fundamental for people with diabetes, there is developing acknowledgment of the significance of overseeing diabetes normally through way of life alterations and comprehensive methodologies. Natural diabetes management has the potential to empower individuals to take control of their health and provide them with significant advantages. Natural diabetes management is essential for the following important reasons:

Control of Blood Sugar: Controlling blood sugar levels requires natural management strategies like eating a healthy diet and getting more exercise. People can better control their blood sugar levels and lower their risk of hyperglycemia (high blood sugar) and hypoglycemia (low blood sugar) by choosing healthy foods and exercising regularly. Maintaining overall health and preventing complications necessitate stable blood sugar control.

Reduced Need for Medication: Naturally managing diabetes can frequently reduce medication dependence. People may be able to increase their insulin sensitivity by making changes to their lifestyle. This will make it easier for their bodies to use the insulin they make or inject. Under the supervision of a medical professional, this may lead to lower medication doses or even the possibility of quitting some medications altogether. The financial burden and overall health of a person can both benefit from lowering their medication dependence.

Controlling your weight: Normal administration of diabetes frequently includes embracing a solid eating regimen and expanding actual work, which can add to weight the board or weight reduction. Corpulence is a critical gamble factor for creating type 2 diabetes and can compound the condition in people previously determined to have diabetes. A person's insulin sensitivity, blood sugar control, and risk of diabetes complications can all be improved and reduced by maintaining a healthy weight.

Health of the Heart: Diabetes is strongly associated with an increased risk of cardiovascular conditions like stroke and heart disease. Overseeing diabetes normally through way of life adjustments can fundamentally decrease the gamble of cardiovascular difficulties. Along with regular exercise, a healthy diet rich in nutrient-dense foods like fruits, vegetables, whole grains, and lean proteins can assist in lowering cholesterol levels, lowering blood pressure, and preserving overall cardiovascular health.

Preventing Complications in the Long Run: Legitimate administration of diabetes assumes a critical part in forestalling or deferring the beginning of long haul entanglements related with the condition. Over time, high blood sugar levels can cause damage to a number of the body's organs and systems, such as the heart, blood vessels, kidneys, eyes, and nerves. People with diabetes can better control their blood sugar levels and lower their risk of complications like diabetic retinopathy, diabetic neuropathy, kidney disease, and cardiovascular diseases by naturally managing their diabetes.

Overall happiness: A holistic approach to health that goes beyond blood sugar control is part of natural diabetes management. Way of life changes, like a nutritious eating routine, ordinary activity, stress decrease strategies, and quality rest, add to in general prosperity. The levels of energy, mood, mental health, and general vitality are all positively impacted by these lifestyle factors. Diabetes patients can improve their quality of life by taking care of their overall health.

Self-management and empowerment: Natural diabetes management gives people the ability to take control of their health and well-being. By embracing sound propensities and pursuing informed decisions, people can foster a feeling of command over their condition. Regular administration procedures energize self-observing, self-control, and taking care of oneself, encouraging a proactive way to deal with diabetes the board.

In conclusion, natural diabetes management is of the utmost importance to those who suffer from this persistent condition. By executing way of life changes, people can accomplish better glucose control, diminish prescription reliance, oversee weight, work on cardiovascular wellbeing, forestall long haul entanglements, improve generally speaking prosperity, and gain a feeling of strengthening. It is critical to talk with medical care experts for direction and customized exhortation

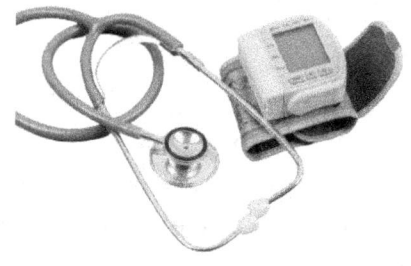

Sugar Level Testing

CHAPTER TWO

MODIFICATIONS TO YOUR LIFESTYLE TO CONTROL DIABETES

Diabetes is a chronic condition that requires a comprehensive management strategy. While drug is in many cases a urgent part, way of life changes assume an essential part in controlling glucose levels and lessening the gamble of difficulties. Changes in one's lifestyle can have a big effect on managing diabetes and overall health. Changes to one's lifestyle that can make a big difference in how well someone manages diabetes:

Smart dieting:

Diabetes management is centered on eating a healthy diet. In order to regulate blood sugar levels and maintain overall health, it requires mindful food choices. The accompanying dietary rules are especially helpful for people with diabetes:

Monitoring of Carbohydrates: Blood sugar control requires careful monitoring and control of carbohydrate intake. Carbs fundamentally affect glucose levels, so it's critical to pick high-fiber, complex carbs, like entire grains, vegetables, organic products, and vegetables, over refined carbs and sweet food sources.

Control of Size: Weight management and blood sugar control are both aided by portion control. A balanced diet requires balancing the portions of various food groups like carbohydrates, proteins, and fats.

Glycemic File: Understanding how certain foods affect blood sugar levels can be made easier by taking into consideration the glycemic index (GI) of those foods. Consuming foods with a low glycemic index (GI) can help keep blood sugar levels stable and reduce spikes.

Healthy Meals: Lean proteins, healthy fats, whole grains, and fruits and vegetables with a lot of fiber help control blood sugar levels and provide essential nutrients.

Ordinary Feast Examples: Blood sugar levels can be kept consistent throughout the day by following regular mealtime routines, such as eating three main meals and including healthy snacks.

Customary Active work:

Active work has various advantages for people with diabetes. It assists in lowering blood sugar levels, increases insulin sensitivity, aids in weight loss, improves cardiovascular health, and enhances well-being in general. Participating in moderate-power oxygen consuming exercises, like lively strolling, cycling, swimming, or moving, for somewhere around 150 minutes of the week is suggested. Furthermore, integrating strength preparing practices something like two days seven days assists work with muscling mass, increment digestion, and further develop insulin awareness.

Controlling your weight:

For diabetes management, it is essential to maintain a healthy weight. Insulin resistance and the likelihood of complications are increased by excess body weight, particularly abdominal fat. A well-balanced diet and regular exercise are essential for achieving and maintaining a healthy weight. In order to effectively manage weight, it can be helpful to set attainable goals, monitor progress, and seek support from healthcare professionals or support groups.

Stress Reduction:

By causing hormonal changes that raise blood glucose levels, chronic stress can have an effect on blood sugar control. Diabetes sufferers need to find healthy ways to deal with stress. Deep breathing exercises, mindfulness exercises, yoga, and other stress-relieving activities, as well as hobbies, can help improve well-being and reduce stress levels.

Normal Glucose Checking:

Ordinary glucose observing is fundamental for diabetes the board. It aids individuals in comprehending how lifestyle choices like diet, exercise, medication, stress, and other factors affect blood sugar levels. Checking gives important data to making fundamental changes and keeping up with ideal glucose control. Medical services experts can direct people on the recurrence and timing of glucose checking.

Quality sleep:

Diabetes management necessitates quality sleep at a sufficient level. Unfortunate rest examples and lack of sleep can influence glucose control and insulin responsiveness. Laying out a steady rest schedule, establishing a helpful rest climate, and pursuing great rest cleanliness routines, for example, restricting caffeine consumption and electronic gadget use before bed, can add to all the more likely rest quality.

Moderation in Alcohol and Quitting Smoking:

Smoking and unreasonable liquor utilization can build the gamble of diabetes .

THE JOB OF DIET IN DIABETES CONTROL

The board Diet assumes a principal part in the administration of diabetes. Pursuing quality food decisions can assist with directing glucose levels, advance weight the board, diminish the gamble of entanglements, and upgrade by and large prosperity. The key to managing diabetes is a diet that is well-balanced and tailored to each person's needs. The following are some important considerations regarding the role that diet plays in diabetes management:

Starch Counting:

Since carbohydrates have the greatest impact on blood sugar levels, it's important to keep an eye on and control how much you eat. In carbohydrate counting, the number of carbohydrates consumed at each meal is tracked and, if necessary, matched with the appropriate insulin dose or medication. This approach assists people with keeping up with stable glucose levels over the course of the day.

GI (glycemic index):

A ranking system known as the glycemic index (GI) indicates how quickly a particular food raises blood sugar levels. Blood sugar spikes can be reduced by choosing low-GI foods, which are digested and absorbed more slowly. High-fiber food varieties, entire grains, vegetables, non-dull vegetables, and most natural products will quite often have a lower GI, pursuing them valuable decisions for people with diabetes.

Control of Size:

In order to control blood sugar levels and encourage weight loss, portion control is essential. Preventing blood sugar swings and excessive calorie intake is made easier by eating in moderation. Working with an enrolled dietitian can give direction on fitting piece sizes and dinner arranging.

Healthy Meals:

Diabetes management necessitates the creation of well-balanced meals that incorporate healthy fats, proteins, and carbohydrates. Proteins can be obtained from lean meats, poultry, fish, tofu, or plant-based sources like beans and lentils. Carbohydrates should come from nutrient-dense sources like whole grains, fruits, vegetables, and legumes. A well-balanced diet should also include healthy fats like olive oil, avocados, nuts, and seeds.

Fiber-Rich Food sources:

Diabetes patients benefit from including foods high in fiber in their diet. The digestion and absorption of carbohydrates is slowed by fiber, which contributes to the stabilization of blood sugar levels. It also helps you feel full, helps you lose weight, and keeps your digestive system healthy. Entire grains, natural products, vegetables, vegetables, and nuts are brilliant wellsprings of dietary fiber.

Sweeteners and sugars:

Overseeing sugar admission is fundamental for diabetes control. It is vital to restrict the utilization of food varieties and refreshments high in added sugars, like sweet beverages, desserts, pastries, and handled food sources. All things considered, people can pick normal sugars with some restraint, like stevia, erythritol, or priest natural product separate, which insignificantly affect glucose levels.

Healthy Consumption:

It is essential to select healthy snacks to prevent fluctuations in blood sugar and maintain energy levels throughout the day. Bites ought to in a perfect world incorporate a blend of starches, proteins, and sound fats. Models incorporate a modest bunch of nuts, Greek yogurt, crude vegetables with hummus, or a little piece of natural product with nut margarine.

Fluids Taken in:

Hydration is essential for diabetes management and overall health. It is essential to drink enough water throughout the day to keep hydrated properly. Sweet beverages, natural product squeezes, and improved refreshments ought to be restricted or stayed away from because of their effect on glucose levels.

Normal Feast Examples:

Blood sugar levels can be maintained consistently by planning meals in a consistent manner. It is essential to consume well-balanced meals on a regular basis and to avoid skipping meals. Having three main meals spread out throughout the day and including healthy snacks helps keep blood sugar levels in check and prevents overeating.

COMING UP WITH A BALANCED MEAL PLAN

A well-balanced meal plan is an essential component of a healthy lifestyle, particularly for diabetics. A well-thought-out and well-balanced diet can help keep blood sugar levels in check, encourage weight loss, supply necessary nutrients, and lower the risk of complications. Making a decent feast plan includes considering segment sizes, nutritional categories, supplement piece, and individual inclinations. When making a meal plan that is balanced, the following are some important things to keep in mind:

Comprehension of Macronutrients:

The three main nutrients in our diet are called macronutrients. fats, proteins, and carbohydrates Each macronutrient assumes a particular part in the body and ought to be remembered for fitting extents in a fair dinner plan.

Carbohydrates: Carbs are the essential wellspring of energy and greatestly affect glucose levels. Counting complex carbs, like entire grains, vegetables, organic products, and vegetables, is gainful as they give fundamental fiber, nutrients, and minerals. For blood sugar control, carbohydrate intake must be monitored, and portion sizes should be carefully considered.

Proteins: Proteins are necessary for supporting the immune system, building and repairing tissues, and regulating blood sugar levels. Lean meats, poultry, fish, eggs, tofu, legumes, and dairy products are all good sources of protein. Remembering protein for every feast can assist with advancing satiety and balance out glucose levels.

Fats: Healthy fats are necessary for the production of hormones, the absorption of nutrients, and the provision of energy. Avocados, olive oil, nuts, seeds, and fatty fish are all good sources of healthy fats. Because they contain a lot of calories, it's important to eat healthy fats in moderation.

Control of Size:

In order to control blood sugar levels and maintain a healthy weight, portion control is essential. Adjusting how much food ate can forestall exorbitant calorie admission and changes in glucose levels. An overall rule is to fill half of the plate with non-dull vegetables, one-quarter with lean protein, and one-quarter with entire grains or bland vegetables. Working with an enrolled dietitian can give customized direction on proper part estimates.

Get your fill of non-starchy vegetables:

Vegetables that aren't starchy are high in fiber, vitamins, and minerals and low in calories and carbs. They can be consumed in large quantities and have little effect on blood sugar levels. A variety of non-starchy vegetables, like leafy greens, broccoli, cauliflower, peppers, zucchini, and cucumbers, can help fill you up and make you feel fuller.

Whole grains and foods high in fiber:

Whole grains are preferable to refined grains because they contain more vitamins, minerals, and fiber. Foods high in fiber help to control blood sugar levels, make digestion easier, and make you feel fuller longer. Oats, whole grain pasta, whole wheat bread, and brown rice are all examples of whole grains. Try to consume at least half of your grains as whole grains.

Lean Proteins:

Lean protein is important for controlling blood sugar and overall health. Saturated fats and calories are lower in lean proteins. Great decisions incorporate skinless poultry, fish, lean cuts of meat, tofu, tempeh, vegetables, and low-fat dairy items. Throughout the day, consuming a variety of proteins helps satisfy nutritional requirements and supplies essential amino acids.

Sound Fats With some restraint:

Sound fats, like monounsaturated and polyunsaturated fats, are fundamental for the body. They aid in the supply of fat-soluble vitamins and essential fatty acids. Avocados, olive oil, nuts, seeds, and fatty fish are all good sources of healthy fats. However, due to their high calorie content, it is essential to consume healthy fats in moderation.

Integrating exercise into your daily routine is an essential component of diabetes management and overall health promotion. Improve insulin sensitivity, manage weight, improve cardiovascular health, and lower the risk of complications are all benefits of regular physical activity. Diabetes patients may find it enjoyable and beneficial to incorporate exercise into their daily routine. When incorporating exercise into your routine, there are a few important things to keep in mind:

Speak with a Medical Professional:

Prior to beginning any activity program, it's vital to talk with a medical care proficient, particularly on the off chance that you have previous ailments. They can give customized direction and suggest proper activities in view of your wellness level, generally wellbeing, and any likely dangers or limits.

Choose things you like to do:

To keep up with long haul adherence to a work-out everyday practice, picking exercises that you enjoy is fundamental. Finding activities that you find enjoyable and fulfilling will make it easier to incorporate exercise into your daily life, whether you choose to walk, jog, swim, dance, yoga, or play a sport.

Set attainable goals:

Defining reasonable objectives is pivotal to remain inspired and track progress. Start with small, doable objectives and gradually increase your workout intensity, duration, or frequency. For instance, plan to stroll for 30 minutes, three times each week, and continuously increment the time or distance as you become more agreeable.

Try a Wide Range of Exercises:

Engaging various muscle groups, preventing boredom, and challenging your body are all benefits of incorporating a variety of exercises into your routine. Incorporate a mix of oxygen consuming activities (like energetic strolling, running, or cycling) to work on cardiovascular wellness, strength preparing works out (utilizing loads or obstruction groups) to fabricate bulk and further develop digestion, and adaptability works out (like yoga or extending) to further develop scope of movement and forestall wounds.

Keep an eye on your blood sugar levels:

If you are taking insulin or any medications that have the potential to affect blood sugar, it is critical to keep an eye on your blood sugar levels before, during, and after exercise. Assuming your glucose levels are excessively high or excessively low, it could be important to change your food admission, insulin portions, or medicine timing. For safe and effective exercise, regular monitoring and communication with your healthcare team are essential.

Begin Gradually and Progress Steadily:

It's important to start slowly and gradually increase the intensity and duration of your workouts if you're new to exercise or haven't been active in a while. This permits your body to adjust and decreases the gamble of wounds or extreme weariness. Think about starting with short, low-impact workouts and gradually progressing to longer, more intense workouts over time.

Develop a routine:

When it comes to exercise, consistency is essential. Include regular exercise sessions in your weekly routine to make it a habit. Stick with the time of day that works best for you. Just like with any other important appointment or commitment, exercise should be prioritized.

Observe and adjust:

Focus on how your body answers work out. During and after physical activity, keep an eye on your energy levels, blood sugar responses, and any symptoms you may have. You can use this information to make any necessary adjustments to your exercise routine, such as adjusting the intensity, duration, or timing of your workouts to better control your blood sugar.

Keep hydrated:

Make sure to remain hydrated previously, during, and after work out. Hydrate consistently to forestall parchedness, particularly in blistering climate or during extreme exercises. Unless absolutely necessary to treat low blood sugar, avoid sports drinks and beverages high in sugar.

Seek Companions and Support:

When it comes to sticking to a workout schedule, having support and someone to hold you accountable can be very helpful. Consider practicing with a companion or joining a wellness gathering or class. Offering your objectives and progress to others can give inspiration, and consolation to you.

THE EXECUTIVES STRATEGIES FOR DIABETES CONTROL

Overseeing pressure is critical for people with diabetes as constant pressure can affect glucose levels and generally wellbeing. Stress causes the release of hormones like cortisol and adrenaline, which can make insulin work less effectively and raise blood glucose levels. Diabetics can better manage their condition and improve their overall well-being by incorporating stress management strategies into their daily lives. Here are some successful treasures of executives methods for diabetes control:

Actual work:

Not only is regular exercise good for controlling blood sugar, but it's also a great way to manage stress. Endorphins, which are naturally occurring chemicals that improve mood and aid in stress reduction and relaxation, are released during exercise. On most days of the week, aim for at least 30 minutes of moderate-intensity aerobic activity, such as brisk walking, swimming, cycling, or dancing. Stress can be relieved throughout the day by engaging in even short bursts of activity, such as taking the stairs or stretching breaks.

Exercises in Deep Breathing:

For calming the mind and easing stress, deep breathing exercises are effective yet simple methods. Take slow, deep breaths through your mouth while sitting or lying down in a comfortable position. Keep your attention on your breath and, with each breath, picture positive energy entering your body and stress leaving it. You can practice deep breathing wherever and whenever you feel overwhelmed or stressed.

Mindfulness and meditation:

Relaxation, anxiety reduction, and self-awareness are all aided by mindfulness and meditation practices. Track down a peaceful and agreeable space, sit in a casual position, and concentrate on the current second. You can use guided meditation apps or recordings, focus on your breath, or repeat a soothing word or phrase. Mindfulness is the practice of not judging your thoughts, feelings, or sensations. Meditating and practicing mindfulness on a regular basis can assist in stress management and enhance emotional well-being.

Tai Chi and yoga:

Yoga and Kendo are mind-body rehearses that consolidate actual development, profound breathing, and reflection. These practices advance unwinding, further develop adaptability, improve balance, and lessen pressure. Tai Chi is characterized by slow, fluid movements, whereas yoga consists of gentle stretching exercises and poses. Both activities can be practiced in classes or at home using online resources and can be modified to suit various fitness levels and abilities.

Social Assistance:

Emotional relief and assistance managing stress can be obtained by seeking support from friends, family, or support groups.

Interfacing with other people who have comparative encounters can offer a feeling of having a place, understanding, and support. Discuss your thoughts and worries with believed people, join diabetes support gatherings or online networks, or consider conversing with a guide or advisor who has practical experience in diabetes-related pressure the board.

Using time productively:

By giving your day-to-day life structure and organization, effective time management can help you feel less stressed. Set attainable objectives, prioritize tasks and responsibilities, and divide them into manageable chunks. When possible, learn to delegate tasks and decline additional commitments that could overwhelm you. Putting together a schedule or to-do list can help you feel more in control and less overwhelmed.

Methods of Relaxation:

Stress can be reduced by incorporating relaxation techniques into your daily routine. Attempt methods like moderate muscle unwinding, where you tense and delivery each muscle gathering to advance physical and mental unwinding. Warm baths, calming music, hobbies or creative pursuits, and aromatherapy with essential oils known for their ability to alleviate stress are additional methods of relaxation.

Healthy habits for life:

Keeping a solid way of life can by implication assist with overseeing pressure. To ensure your mental and physical health, get enough sleep. Eat a well-balanced diet because certain nutrients, like B vitamins and omega-3 fatty acids, can help your brain stay healthy and help you feel less stressed. Drinking alcohol and caffeine should be avoided as much as possible.

CHAPTER THREE

THE POWER OF NATURAL FOODS

Whole foods, also known as natural foods, are low in processing and have numerous health advantages. Natural foods are a powerful way to improve your overall health, manage chronic conditions like diabetes, and feel better overall. Natural foods have a tremendous amount of power for the following reasons:

Supplement Thickness:

Vitamins, minerals, antioxidants, dietary fiber, and other vital nutrients are abundant in natural foods. Natural foods provide a concentrated dose of nourishment in every bite, in contrast to processed foods, which frequently lack these essential nutrients. Fruits and vegetables, for instance, are loaded with vitamins and minerals that help the body's immune system function properly, guard against long-term illnesses, and promote optimal health.

A Lot Of Fiber:

Natural foods are excellent sources of dietary fiber, which is an essential component of a healthy diet. Fiber helps with digestion, keeps blood sugar levels in check, makes you feel full, and is good for your heart. Normal food varieties like entire grains, vegetables, organic products, and vegetables are plentiful in fiber, making them fundamental for keeping a decent and nutritious eating routine.

Antioxidant-Rich:

Antioxidants are abundant in natural foods, particularly fruits, vegetables, nuts, and seeds. Cells are shielded from harm by free radicals, harmful molecules, thanks to antioxidants. By killing free revolutionaries, cell reinforcements diminish the gamble of persistent infections like coronary illness, disease, and neurodegenerative problems. Include a wide range of colorful fruits and vegetables in your diet to get a healthy dose of antioxidants.

Glucose Control:

For people with diabetes, regular food sources assume a fundamental part in overseeing glucose levels. When compared to processed foods, whole foods, particularly those with complex carbohydrates like whole grains, legumes, and vegetables, have a lower glycemic index. As a result, they are digested and absorbed more slowly, preventing abrupt spikes in blood sugar levels. This results in a gradual release of glucose into the bloodstream. Natural foods can help maintain stable blood sugar levels and reduce the need for excessive insulin or medication in a diabetes-friendly diet.

wholesome fats:

Natural foods contain healthy fats, which are necessary for good health. Monounsaturated and polyunsaturated fats, including omega-3 fatty acids, are abundant in avocados, nuts, seeds, and fatty fish. These fats support cerebrum wellbeing, diminish irritation, advance heart wellbeing, and help in the assimilation of fat-dissolvable nutrients. Natural sources of healthy fats can help you feel better all around and lower your risk of chronic diseases.

Reduced Exposure to Chemicals:

Preservatives, artificial additives, and chemicals that are frequently found in processed foods are not present in natural foods. By picking normal food sources, you lessen your openness to possibly hurtful substances, including fake sugars, high-fructose corn syrup, and trans fats. Keeping your intake of these additives to a minimum can benefit your health and lower the likelihood of negative effects.

Worked on Stomach related Wellbeing:

Due to their high fiber content, natural foods are beneficial to digestive health. Fiber advances standard solid discharges, forestalls stoppage, and supports a sound stomach microbiome. Improved digestion, enhanced immune function, and decreased inflammation are all linked to a gut microbiome that is both diverse and balanced. Natural foods like whole grains, legumes, fruits, and vegetables help your digestive system stay healthy.

Overall Happiness:

Natural foods have a positive effect on one's overall health. A supplement thick eating regimen gives the essential fuel to ideal physical and mental capability, further developing energy levels, temperament, and mental capacities. You are giving yourself the best chance to thrive and live a high quality of life by feeding your body natural, nutritious foods.

INVESTIGATING DIABETES

Accommodating Food varieties,

Overseeing diabetes requires cautious consideration regarding one's eating routine. Controlling blood sugar levels and maintaining overall health are both greatly aided by choosing healthy foods. Fortunately, there is a wide selection of delicious and nutritious diabetes-friendly foods available. We'll look at some of these foods and what they can do for diabetics in this article.

Vegetables That Aren't Starchy:

Non-bland vegetables are loaded with fundamental supplements, high in fiber, and have a low glycemic record, settling on them a great decision for individuals with diabetes. Instances of non-dull vegetables incorporate mixed greens (spinach, kale), broccoli, cauliflower, peppers, zucchini, and asparagus. These vegetables can be enjoyed in a variety of ways, including roasted, stir-fried, and salads.

Whole Cereals:

For diabetes management, whole grains over refined grains are essential. There is more fiber, vitamins, and minerals in whole grains like brown rice, quinoa, oats, and whole wheat bread or pasta. They likewise have a lower glycemic file, bringing about a more slow ascent in glucose levels. Integrating entire grains into dinners gives supported energy and advances stomach related wellbeing.

Sources of Lean Proteins:

Lean protein helps maintain normal blood sugar levels and supplies essential nutrients. Select lean sources like skinless poultry, fish, tofu, eggs, and vegetables like lentils and beans. These protein sources are low in soaked fats and give a variety of nutrients and minerals that help in general wellbeing.

wholesome fats:

Not all fats are harmful, contrary to popular belief. Solid fats, like those tracked down in avocados, nuts, seeds, and olive oil, are gainful for people with diabetes. These fats are good for your heart, make you feel full, and give you energy slowly and steadily. However, due to their high calorie content, it is essential to consume healthy fats in moderation.

Dairy With Low Fat:

When consumed in moderation and in low- or no-fat versions, dairy products can be a part of a diabetes-friendly diet. Low-fat milk, yogurt, and curds are rich wellsprings of calcium, protein, and vitamin D. These supplements are essential for keeping up with bone wellbeing and supporting by and large prosperity.

Berries:

Vitamins, fiber, and antioxidants abound in berries like strawberries, blueberries, and raspberries. They are a great choice for satisfying your sweet tooth without significantly raising blood sugar levels because they have a glycemic index that is lower than that of other fruits. Appreciate berries as a tidbit, add them to smoothies, or use them to finish off your morning oats or yogurt.

Spices and Herbs:

Involving spices and flavors in your cooking is a fantastic method for adding flavor without depending on unnecessary measures of salt, sugar, or undesirable toppings. The anti-inflammatory properties of cinnamon, turmeric, ginger, garlic, and oregano may help regulate blood sugar levels. Try different spices and herbs to make your food taste better and get the most out of their potential health benefits.

Important aspects of diabetes management include portion control and carbohydrate monitoring. A registered dietitian or other healthcare professional should be consulted before developing a bespoke meal plan that meets your specific requirements.

In conclusion, trying foods that are good for diabetes can show you a lot of delicious and healthy options. Non-dull vegetables, entire grains, lean proteins, sound fats, low-fat dairy, berries, and spices/flavors are only a couple of instances of the numerous decisions accessible. People with diabetes can better manage their condition and improve their overall health and well-being by making smart food choices and eating a balanced diet.

SUPER FOODS FOR BLOOD SUGAR REGULATION

It is essential for people with diabetes, those attempting to prevent diabetes, and those managing their overall health to maintain stable blood sugar levels. Including superfoods in your diet can help you naturally control your blood sugar levels in a great way. Due to their low glycemic index and abundance of essential nutrients, antioxidants, and fiber, superfoods are ideal for maintaining stable blood sugar levels. In this article, we will investigate some superfoods that can support glucose guideline.

Seeds Of Chia:

Chia seeds are tiny nutritional powerhouses. They are an excellent source of protein, fiber, and omega-3 fatty acids. The high fiber content in chia seeds dials back processing and forestalls glucose spikes. Additionally, chia seeds have the ability to take in water and form a gel-like substance in the stomach, which helps people feel fuller and prevents them from overeating. Chia seeds can be added to oatmeal, smoothies, yogurt, and baking recipes as an alternative to eggs.

Leafy Vegetables:

Vitamins, minerals, and antioxidants abound in leafy greens like Swiss chard, spinach, and kale. They are high in fiber and contain few calories and carbohydrates. The high fiber content guides in dialing back the processing and retention of sugars in the circulation system. Additionally, leafy greens contain magnesium, which contributes to insulin sensitivity. A great way to include leafy greens in your diet is by adding them to salads, stir-fries, or smoothies.

Cinnamon:

It has been demonstrated that cinnamon, a spice, helps regulate blood sugar levels. It has substances that can help cells absorb glucose from the bloodstream by acting like insulin. Cinnamon has also been shown to increase insulin sensitivity and lower fasting blood sugar levels. To reap its potential benefits, sprinkle cinnamon on oatmeal, yogurt, or bake recipes.

Turmeric:

Curcumin, a component in turmeric that has been linked to improved blood sugar control, is what gives it its vibrant yellow color. Curcumin may improve insulin sensitivity and reduce insulin resistance by acting as an anti-inflammatory. Adding turmeric to curries, broiled vegetables, or smoothies could upgrade the flavor at any point as well as give potential glucose controlling advantages.

Berries:

Strawberries, blueberries, and raspberries are examples of berries that are low in sugar but high in fiber and antioxidants. They have a low glycemic record, meaning they cause a more slow ascent in glucose levels contrasted with different natural products. Berries contain fiber, which slows digestion and prevents sudden spikes in blood sugar. Berries can be consumed raw, blended into smoothies, or topped with yogurt or oatmeal.

Quinoa:

Quinoa is a grain that doesn't contain gluten and has a lot of protein, fiber, and vitamins and minerals. It can help maintain blood sugar levels and has a low glycemic index. Quinoa is a flexible fixing that can be utilized as a substitute for rice or added to plates of mixed greens, soups, and sautés.

Nuts and Seeds:

Healthy fats, protein, and fiber are abundant in nuts and seeds like pumpkin seeds, flaxseeds, almonds, and walnuts. The combination of these nutrients aids in reducing the rate at which sugars enter the bloodstream and keeps blood sugar levels stable. Nuts and seeds can also be enjoyed as a snack or added to salads and smoothies for a satisfying crunch.

Integrating these super foods into your eating routine can add to more readily glucose guideline. Nevertheless, it is essential to keep in mind that moderation and portion control are essenti

HERBAL REMEDIES AND SUPPLEMENTS FOR DIABETES MANAGEMENT

Some people with diabetes look into herbal remedies and supplements as complementary approaches to managing their condition. Consult a registered dietitian or other healthcare professional to create a well-balanced meal plan that meets your individual requirements. There are a number of herbs and supplements that have demonstrated promise in supporting blood sugar regulation and overall diabetes management, despite the fact that it is essential to consult a healthcare professional before incorporating any new remedies or supplements into your routine. We'll look at some of these supplements and herbal remedies in this article.

Cinnamon:

A well-known spice with the potential to lower blood sugar is cinnamon. It contains substances that may help cells better absorb glucose from the bloodstream and increase insulin sensitivity. Cinnamon supplementation has been shown in a number of studies to improve fasting blood sugar levels and lower HbA1c levels, which are long-term indicators of blood sugar control. It very well may be consumed in powder structure or taken as an enhancement, however it's essential to pick excellent sources and talk with a medical care proficient for legitimate dose direction.

Gymnema Sylvestre:

Gymnema Sylvestre is a spice local to India and has been generally utilized in Ayurvedic medication to help diabetes the board. It is thought to lower blood sugar levels by increasing insulin production and inhibiting sugar absorption in the intestine. Some examination proposes that Gymnema Sylvestre might assist with lessening fasting glucose levels and further develop HbA1c levels. Nonetheless, more examinations are expected to completely grasp its viability and decide suitable doses.

Fenugreek:

Traditional medicine often uses fenugreek seeds to help control blood sugar. They are high in fiber and contain substances that may increase insulin sensitivity and secretion. Studies have demonstrated the way that fenugreek supplementation can prompt superior fasting glucose levels and glucose resilience in people with diabetes. Fenugreek can be consumed as a zest or taken in case structure, however it's essential to talk with a medical care proficient for fitting dosing and to screen for any expected collaborations with prescriptions.

Acid Alpha-Lipoic:

The body naturally produces powerful antioxidant called alpha-lipoic acid (ALA). It has been studied to see if it could help manage diabetes. Reduced oxidative stress, increased insulin sensitivity, and improved peripheral neuropathy symptoms in diabetics have all been shown to benefit from ALA. It is available as a dietary supplement; however, it is essential to consult a medical professional regarding the appropriate dosage and potential side effects.

Chromium:

The metabolism of glucose and insulin both require chromium, a mineral. A few examinations propose that chromium supplementation might assist further develop insulin responsiveness and glucose control in people with diabetes. But more research is needed to figure out the best doses and how it works over time. Before beginning chromium supplementation, it is essential to consult a medical professional due to the risk of adverse effects from excessive consumption.

Sweet Melon:

Traditional medicine has long used bitter melon, a tropical fruit, to help control blood sugar. It contains substances that may help lower blood sugar levels and mimic the effects of insulin. Taking a bitter melon supplement has been shown in some studies to improve blood sugar levels during and after meals. Bitter melon can be consumed in juice, tea, or capsules, but it is important to talk to a doctor about the right dosage and keep an eye out for any possible interactions or side effects.

It is essential to keep in mind that, despite the fact that these herbal remedies and supplements may have potential advantages, they should not be used in place of traditional medical treatment or lifestyle changes for the management of diabetes. Before incorporating any new treatments or supplements into your routine, it is important to talk to a doctor or registered dietitian. They can help keep track of your progress and offer advice on the right dosages and potential drug interactions.

The benefits of foods high in fiber for diabetes management A healthy diet is essential for diabetes management and overall well-being. It is wise to include foods high in fiber in your diet if you want to control your diabetes. For diabetics, fiber is an important part of a well-balanced diet that has many benefits. In this article, we will investigate the advantages of fiber-rich food varieties and how they can uphold diabetes control.

Glucose Guideline:

Fiber-rich foods' ability to regulate blood sugar levels is one of their primary diabetes management benefits. Solvent fiber, found in food varieties like oats, vegetables, and organic products, dials back the processing and retention of starches, prompting a more continuous ascent in glucose levels after a dinner. This can assist with forestalling fast spikes and dunks in glucose, advancing more steady glucose command over the long run.

Further developed Insulin Awareness:

Foods high in fiber have been linked to increased insulin sensitivity. Insulin is the chemical liable for managing glucose levels, and people with diabetes frequently battle with insulin opposition. A diet high in fiber has been shown to increase insulin sensitivity, allowing cells to respond to insulin more effectively and contributing to proper blood sugar control.

Weight The executives:

For diabetes management, maintaining a healthy weight is essential, and fiber-rich foods can assist in this regard. Foods with a lot of fiber tend to be more filling, so people feel fuller longer and eat fewer calories. You can help prevent overeating and promote weight management by including whole grains, vegetables, and legumes in your diet. You can also feel full for longer periods of time.

Health of the Heart:

Diabetes is associated with an increased risk of cardiovascular problems. Fiber-rich food varieties can add to heart wellbeing by bringing down cholesterol levels. Low-density lipoprotein (LDL) cholesterol, also known as "bad" cholesterol, is reduced specifically by soluble fiber. You can support a healthy heart and lower your risk of cardiovascular diseases linked to diabetes by including foods high in fiber in your diet.

Stomach related Wellbeing:

Fiber is fundamental for keeping a solid stomach related framework. It adds mass to the stool, advances standard defecations, and forestalls stoppage, a typical issue for people with diabetes. You can support proper digestion and alleviate gastrointestinal discomfort by consuming sufficient amounts of fiber from whole grains, fruits, vegetables, and legumes.

Long haul Diabetes The board:

Reliably remembering fiber-rich food sources for your eating routine can add to long haul diabetes the board. By zeroing in on entire food sources and keeping away from handled and refined choices, you can guarantee a higher admission of fiber. This strategy helps manage diabetes-related complications over time, supports stable blood sugar levels, and provides a more balanced nutrient profile.

It is essential to gradually incorporate fiber-rich foods into your diet and to consume more water in addition to fiber. This ensures optimal benefits and helps prevent discomfort in the digestive tract. Also, it's a good idea to talk to a registered dietitian or other health care professional about creating a custom meal plan that fits your needs and tastes.

In conclusion, diabetics can benefit from a variety of foods high in fiber. From glucose guideline and further developed insulin aversion to weight the executives, cardiovascular wellbeing, and stomach related prosperity, the consideration of fiber-rich food varieties can uphold generally diabetes control. You can create a balanced diet that promotes stable blood sugar levels, lowers the risk of complications, and improves your overall health and well-being by including whole grains, legumes, fruits, vegetables, and other fiber-rich foods in your meals.

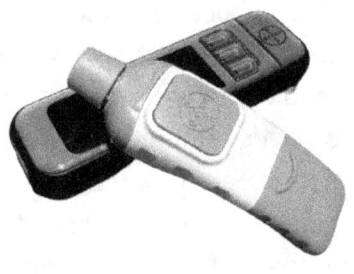

Sugar Level Strip

CHAPTER FOUR

THE EFFECT F SUGAR AND CARBS ON DIABETES

Diabetes is an ongoing metabolic problem described by high glucose levels. Diabetes is becoming more common all over the world, and lifestyle factors like diet play a significant role in its development. Sugar and carbohydrates are frequently cited as major contributors to the development of diabetes and its management. The relationship between dietary choices and the risk of developing and managing diabetes is shed light on in this article, which examines the impact of sugar and carbohydrates on diabetes.

The Job Of Sugar In Diabetes

Diabetes has been linked to sugar, particularly refined sugars like table sugar (sucrose) and high-fructose corn syrup. At the point when we consume sugar, it is quickly separated into glucose, prompting a spike in glucose levels. Accordingly, the pancreas discharges insulin, a chemical that helps transport glucose into cells for energy creation. However, insulin resistance—a condition in which cells become less responsive to insulin's action—can develop over time from an excessive sugar intake.

Insulin opposition is a forerunner to type 2 diabetes, the most well-known type of diabetes. It makes it harder for the body to effectively control blood sugar levels. High sugar consumption likewise adds to corpulence, another gamble factor for type 2 diabetes. In addition, eating too much sugar can make you gain weight, which makes insulin resistance worse and makes you more likely to get diabetes.

The Importance of Carbohydrates in Diabetes Management The body's primary energy source is carbohydrates. During digestion, they are broken down into glucose, which enters the bloodstream and raises blood sugar levels. The effects of various types of carbohydrates on blood sugar levels vary. Basic starches, tracked down in sweet food varieties, are quickly processed and cause a sharp spike in glucose levels. Because they take longer to digest, complex carbohydrates like whole grains, legumes, and vegetables raise blood sugar levels more gradually.

Controlling one's carbohydrate intake is essential for diabetes patients to achieve steady blood sugar levels. To assist diabetics in making informed dietary choices, carbohydrate counting is frequently recommended. Controlling blood sugar levels and reducing medication use can be accomplished by monitoring the type and quantity of carbohydrates consumed.

The effect of sugar and carbs on diabetes is huge. Consuming an excessive amount of sugar can contribute to insulin resistance and raise the risk of type 2 diabetes. People who are at risk for developing diabetes or who have already been diagnosed with the disease need to keep an eye on their sugar intake and cut back on it. Also, overseeing starch admission, especially by zeroing in on complex carbs, can assist people with diabetes keep up with stable glucose levels. Individuals can reduce their risk of developing diabetes and effectively manage their condition, thereby enhancing their overall health and well-being, by adopting a diet that is well-balanced and nutritious.

Understanding how sugar affects blood sugar levels Sugar is a common ingredient in a wide range of foods and beverages. Sugar is broken down into glucose, a simple sugar that is the body's primary energy source, through digestion when we consume it. However, consuming an excessive amount of sugar can result in a rapid rise in blood sugar levels. The purpose of this article is to investigate the mechanisms by which sugar affects blood sugar levels and the potential health effects of eating a lot of sugar.

The Glycemic List and Sugar

A scale called the glycemic index (GI) measures how quickly and significantly a specific food raises blood sugar levels. Blood sugar levels quickly rise in response to foods with a high GI, such as sugary beverages, sweets, and processed carbohydrates. Conversely, food varieties with a low GI, like entire grains, vegetables, and non-dull vegetables, lead to an increasingly slow continuous ascent in glucose levels.

Consuming a lot of sugar can make the body use up too much glucose, which can cause blood sugar levels to rise quickly. Insulin, a hormone that helps transport glucose from the bloodstream into cells, is released as a response by the pancreas. This instrument manages glucose levels and guarantee sufficient energy supply to the body's cells. However, insulin resistance, a condition in which the cells become less responsive to insulin's action, can develop over time from an excessive sugar intake. Type 2 diabetes is characterized by persistently elevated blood sugar levels due to this resistance.

Sugar And Its Effects On Health

High sugar admission influences glucose levels as well as has different wellbeing suggestions. Because the body converts excess sugar into fat and stores it, it contributes to obesity. Heftiness, thus, builds the gamble of creating insulin opposition and type 2 diabetes.

A diet high in sugar has also been linked to a higher risk of cardiovascular diseases like hypertension and heart disease. Consuming a lot of sugar can raise triglyceride levels, lower HDL (the good cholesterol) levels, and raise LDL (the bad cholesterol) levels. These progressions in lipid profiles can add to the advancement of atherosclerosis and increment the gamble of heart-related difficulties.

Additionally, dental issues can result from excessive sugary food and beverage consumption. Sugar is the food for bacteria in the mouth, which produce acids that can damage tooth enamel and cause tooth decay.

Understanding the impacts of sugar on glucose levels is urgent for keeping up with generally wellbeing and prosperity. Consuming an excessive amount of sugar can quickly raise blood sugar levels, which can lead to potential health issues like insulin resistance, obesity, cardiovascular disease, and dental issues. People can maintain stable blood sugar levels and lower their risk of developing chronic conditions by being mindful of their sugar intake and choosing healthier options like whole foods and natural sweeteners. Better health outcomes and a more sustainable and well-balanced lifestyle can be achieved by balancing one's diet, reducing added sugars, and making well-informed dietary choices.

THE GLYCEMIC LIST AND ITS IMPORTANCE

The glycemic record (GI) is an action that positions starches in light of their impact on glucose levels. It gives significant experiences into what various food varieties mean for our blood glucose reaction. The GI has received a lot of attention in the nutrition field and is now a useful tool for people who want to control their blood sugar levels, improve their athletic performance, and make better food choices. This article means to investigate the glycemic record and its importance, revealing insight into its applications, restrictions, and expected benefits for in general wellbeing.

Understanding the Glycemic Index:

The glycemic record positions starches on a scale from 0 to 100 in light of how rapidly they raise glucose levels contrasted with a reference food, normally unadulterated glucose or white bread. Food sources with a high GI score, ordinarily over 70, are immediately processed and retained, causing a fast expansion in glucose levels. Contrarily, foods with a low GI score—typically below 55—are absorbed and digested more slowly, resulting in a more gradual rise in blood sugar.

The Glycemic Index's Importance

Individuals with specific dietary requirements or health conditions like diabetes, insulin resistance, and metabolic syndrome can benefit from the information provided by the glycemic index. People can better control their blood sugar levels by knowing what foods have a GI. Blood sugar fluctuations can be reduced by choosing foods with a lower GI. This is especially important for diabetics who need to keep their glucose levels stable.

Athletes and other people looking to improve their performance can also benefit from the glycemic index. Consuming carbs with a moderate to high GI previously or during activity can give a speedy wellspring of energy. Conversely, post-exercise carbohydrate consumption with a low GI can aid in glycogen replenishment and recovery.

The glycemic index can help with weight management in addition to controlling blood sugar and improving athletic performance. People are less likely to overeat or snack on high-sugar foods because foods with a lower GI tend to make them feel fuller for longer periods of time. This can be especially gainful for those hoping to get more fit or keep a sound body weight.

limitations and considerations:

The glycemic index is a useful tool, but it has some restrictions. The ripeness, cooking methods, and food combinations of a food can all have an impact on its GI. Also, the GI doesn't take into account how much food you eat, which can affect how your blood sugar reacts. When choosing a diet, it's important to think about the diet's overall quality as well as the GI.

The glycemic index is a useful tool for understanding how carbohydrates influence blood sugar levels. It is useful for diabetics, athletes looking to improve their performance, and overweight people trying to control their weight. People can help regulate blood sugar levels, increase satiety, and make better food choices by eating foods with a low glycemic index (GI). However, it is essential to take into account the limitations of the glycemic index and incorporate it into a varied and well-balanced diet. By understanding the glycemic file and its importance, people can make proactive strides towards keeping up with ideal wellbeing and prosperity.

Strategies for reducing sugar and refined carbohydrate intake Reducing sugar and carbohydrate intake is crucial for promoting overall health and preventing a variety of chronic diseases, such as diabetes, obesity, and cardiovascular conditions. Notwithstanding, embracing better dietary propensities can be trying because of the predominance of handled food varieties and the habit-forming nature of sugar. The purpose of this article is to offer methods for effectively reducing consumption of sugar and refined carbohydrates, assisting individuals in making changes to their diets that are able to last and enhancing their overall health.

Learn to read food labels and ingredient lists carefully One of the first things you can do to cut back on sugar and refined carbs is to become a careful label reader. Pay close attention to the ingredient lists of packaged foods because sugar can be disguised by many names, including maltose, dextrose, sucrose, and high-fructose corn syrup. Foods with a long list of ingredients should be avoided because they are more likely to contain refined carbohydrates and added sugars. Choose whole foods and products that have been minimally processed.

Pick Entire Food sources

Center around devouring entire, natural food varieties like organic products, vegetables, entire grains, lean proteins, and vegetables. These food sources are normally low in added sugars and high in fiber, nutrients, and minerals. You can significantly reduce your intake of sugar and refined carbohydrates while simultaneously increasing the nutrient density of your diet by substituting whole food alternatives for sugary beverages and processed snacks.

Cook Feasts at Home

Planning feasts at home gives you command over the fixings and cooking strategies. Utilize new fixings and settle on cooking techniques like baking, barbecuing, steaming, or sautéing as opposed to broiling. By preparing your feasts, you can stay away from stowed away sugars and refined carbs ordinarily found in café dishes and bundled accommodation food sources.

Limit Improved Drinks

Sugar-improved refreshments like pop, caffeinated beverages, and natural product juices are significant supporters of unnecessary sugar admission. Select water, natural tea, or unsweetened drinks as choices. For a refreshing beverage with a natural flavor, infuse water with fruits or herbs if you like flavored drinks. Bit by bit decrease your utilization of improved drinks to end the propensity and lower your general sugar admission.

Be aware of condiments and sauces because many of them contain refined carbohydrates and hidden sugars. Look for added sugars on the labels of ketchup, barbecue sauce, salad dressings, and marinades. Consider making your own fixings and dressings utilizing regular sugars like honey, maple syrup, or spices and flavors for some character.

Choose Whole Grain Alternatives Whole grains are preferable to refined grains when selecting grains. Entire grains hold their normal fiber, nutrients, and minerals, pursuing them a better decision. Whole wheat bread, brown rice, quinoa, or other whole grain options can take the place of white bread, white rice, and pasta. These alternatives have a lower glycemic index, so they help keep blood sugar levels in check and give you long-lasting energy.

Practice Portion Control It is essential to practice portion control even when choosing healthier options. Overeating any kind of carbohydrate, refined or not, can cause imbalances in blood sugar and weight gain. Plates and bowls that are smaller can assist in portion control. Center around careful eating, focusing on yearning and totality signals, and appreciating each chomp.

Conclusion: Consuming less refined carbohydrates and sugar is an important part of a healthy diet. People can gradually reduce their intake of refined carbohydrates and added sugars by adopting strategies like reading labels, choosing whole foods, cooking at home, avoiding sweetened beverages, paying attention to condiments, choosing whole grains, and portion control. Changing these things can improve your health as a whole.

Alternatives to sugary treats that are good for you In today's fast-paced world, sugary treats have become an essential part of our diet. Sugar consumption, on the other hand, has been linked to a wide range of health issues, including dental issues, diabetes, and obesity. Fortunately, we can satisfy our sweet tooth cravings with a variety of healthy and delicious alternatives. We can indulge in guilt-free treats without compromising our health by incorporating these options into our daily lives. We'll look at some tempting alternatives to sugary treats that not only taste great but also encourage a healthier lifestyle in this article.

Fruits as Nature's Candy : Nature has given us a wide range of fruits that are not only naturally sweet but also full of vital vitamins, minerals, and dietary fiber. Fruits like mango, watermelon, berries, and pineapple can be enjoyed on their own or in sweet desserts. They give a reviving eruption of pleasantness without the additional sugars tracked down in handled treats. For a refreshing frozen treat, frozen fruits can also be blended into smoothies or pureed to make homemade popsicles.

Dark Chocolate Delights Don't worry if you like chocolate! Dark chocolate, particularly those with a high cocoa content (70 percent or more), can be a healthier choice than white or milk chocolate. Antioxidants are abundant in dark chocolate, which also contains less sugar and unhealthy fats. It has been shown to improve mood, cognitive function, and heart health. Partake in a piece or two of dim chocolate as a periodic treat, or integrate it into recipes, for example, custom made energy bars or trail blend for a liberal yet sustaining nibble.

Nut Butter Heaven: Choose natural nut butters like cashew, almond, or peanut butter instead of spreads that are loaded with unhealthy oils and added sugars. These nut spreads are tasty as well as an extraordinary wellspring of solid fats, protein, and fiber. For a satisfying snack, spread them on whole-grain toast, apple slices, or celery sticks. You can likewise utilize nut spread as a fixing in custom made granola bars, smoothies, or as a plunge for vegetables. Find your favorite guilt-free nut butter recipe by experimenting with various flavors and combinations.

Yogurt Parfaits: A Healthy Alternative to Sugary Desserts Yogurt, especially the Greek variety, is a versatile and healthy option. Greek yogurt is high in probiotics, which aid in gut health, and protein. Layer Greek yogurt, fresh fruits, nuts, and a drizzle of honey or maple syrup for natural sweetness to make a yogurt parfait. Granola or unsweetened coconut flakes can also be sprinkled on top for texture. This brilliant and nutritious sweet can be delighted in as a morning meal choice or as a light and reviving treat over the course of the day.

Enjoying sweet treats can antagonistically affect our wellbeing, however that doesn't mean we need to abandon fulfilling our sweet tooth. We can continue to indulge in delectable and satiating treats without jeopardizing our health by incorporating these nutritious substitutes into our diet. Whether it's the regular pleasantness of natural products, the extravagance of dim chocolate, the richness of nut spread, or the adaptability of yogurt, there are a lot of choices to look over. Therefore, make a conscious effort to embrace these healthier alternatives and begin a journey toward a lifestyle that is more satisfying and well-balanced.

CHAPTER FIVE

CAREFUL EATING AND PART CONTROL

Diabetes is an ongoing condition that influences a great many individuals around the world. It requires cautious administration of glucose levels, which frequently includes rolling out dietary improvements. Mindful eating and portion control are two essential components of a diabetes-friendly diet. People with diabetes can effectively manage their condition and improve their overall well-being by incorporating these practices into their daily lives.

Mindfulness, or being fully present and aware of one's thoughts, feelings, and actions in the present moment, is the foundation of the concept of mindful eating. When applied to eating, it implies giving close consideration to the whole eating experience, including the sight, smell, taste, and surface of food, as well as the body's yearning and completion signals.

Developing a deeper connection with the body's sensations and signals is one of the main benefits of mindful eating for diabetics. By checking out these signs, one can pursue informed decisions about what, when, and the amount to eat. Careful eating likewise advances a feeling of fulfillment and delight from food, prompting a better relationship with eating and diminished chance of indulging.

Slow down and savor each bite in order to practice mindful eating. Enjoy the flavors and textures of the food by taking it all in. Limit interruptions like television, telephones, or PCs during feasts to completely participate in the eating experience. By eating carefully, people with diabetes can more readily check their satiety and forestall unnecessary calorie consumption, which is pivotal for overseeing glucose levels.

One more pivotal part of diabetes the executives is segment control. Preventing spikes in blood sugar and calorie intake is made easier by controlling portion sizes. Because modern food portions have significantly increased over time, it is common for diabetics to struggle with portion sizes. Segment control includes understanding fitting serving sizes and being aware of how much is being consumed.

A supportive device for segment control is utilizing obvious signals and estimating utensils to gauge segment sizes. For instance, a serving of protein (like meat or fish) ought to be generally the size of a deck of cards, while a serving of cooked grains or boring vegetables (like rice or potatoes) ought to be about the size of a tennis ball. Really getting to know these part measures and rehearsing segment control reliably can significantly add to more readily glucose the executives.

In addition, portion control requires awareness of food's calorie and carbohydrate content. Perusing food marks and understanding the nourishing data can assist people with diabetes settle on informed conclusions about segment sizes. It is essential to keep in mind that portion control does not always imply starvation. It's about finding a balance and making decisions that help your health and well-being as a whole.

Mindful eating and portion control can be difficult to implement, especially when confronted with tempting and readily available unhealthy food options. However, there are methods that can help keep these practices going. It can be helpful to avoid impulsive and unhealthy food choices by planning meals in advance, making a shopping list, and having nutritious snacks readily available. Taking part in standard active work can likewise uphold careful eating by expanding familiarity with appetite and satiety signs.

In order to implement strategies for mindful eating and portion control, it can be beneficial to seek support from healthcare professionals, such as diabetes educators or dietitians. They can assist in the creation of individualized meal plans, offer helpful hints, and address specific difficulties associated with diabetes management.

In conclusion, a diabetes-friendly diet must include portion control and mindful eating. Diabetes patients can effectively manage their condition, regulate blood sugar levels, and improve their overall health by practicing mindfulness and being aware of portion sizes. The long-term benefits are well worth the conscious effort and consistent practice required to implement these practices. Mindful eating and portion control can become lifelong habits that contribute to a healthier and happier life with the right tools, support, and dedication.

The importance of mindful eating in diabetes management Millions of people worldwide suffer from diabetes, a chronic condition. To prevent complications and maintain stable blood sugar levels, it requires careful management. Mindful eating is one effective tool that can greatly assist in diabetes management. Being fully present and aware of one's food choices, eating habits, and body's responses to meals is the approach known as mindful eating. Diabetes patients can better control their blood sugar levels and improve their overall well-being by practicing mindful eating.

One of the vital advantages of careful eating for people with diabetes is its capacity to assist with controlling glucose levels. When people eat mindfully, they become more aware of their body's signals of hunger and fullness. They are able to make conscious choices about when to eat, how much to eat, and which foods to eat because of this increased awareness. By eating because of genuine yearning as opposed to close to home or outside prompts, people can all the more likely deal with their glucose levels and forestall superfluous variances.

Mindful eating also helps people learn more about how food choices affect blood sugar levels. Since carbohydrates have the greatest impact on blood sugar levels, diabetics frequently need to keep an eye on their carbohydrate intake. People can learn to appreciate food's nutrient content more deeply through mindfulness and make choices that are in line with their diabetes management goals. While being mindful of portion sizes and carbohydrate counts, they can place a high value on whole, unprocessed foods that are packed with fiber and low in added sugars.

Mindful eating can help people with diabetes control their blood sugar and also help them control their weight, which is important for diabetics. Because excess weight can exacerbate insulin resistance and make managing type 2 diabetes more difficult, many people struggle with weight-related issues. Mindful eating encourages people to eat more slowly, savor each bite, and truly enjoy the eating experience, all of which contribute to a healthier relationship with food. People are more likely to recognize when they are full and avoid overeating when they slow down and pay attention to the body's satiety signals, thereby promoting weight loss or maintenance.

One more part of careful eating that is especially gainful for diabetes the executives is its job in lessening pressure and close to home eating. Because it causes the release of stress hormones, which can lead to an increase in glucose levels, stress can have a significant impact on blood sugar levels. People can help manage their stress levels and prevent emotional eating episodes by practicing mindful eating practices like deep breathing, being present in the moment, and consciously selecting nourishing foods. Stress can have a positive effect on diabetes management if it is addressed at its source and healthier coping mechanisms are found.

In today's fast-paced, food-focused world, practicing mindful eating can be challenging. However, there are methods that can help people adopt and keep up mindful eating habits. For instance, saving devoted dinner times without interruptions like telephones or TV can establish a quiet and centered climate for eating carefully. The mindful eating experience can also be enhanced by planning meals, shopping for nutritious ingredients, and making meals from scratch. In addition, seeking assistance from healthcare professionals, such as diabetes educators or dietitians, can provide helpful direction and motivation for developing mindful eating habits.

As a whole, mindful eating can help diabetics control their blood sugar, control their weight, and improve their overall health. By developing a careful way to deal with food and eating, people can pursue informed decisions about their eating routine, control segment sizes, and better deal with their glucose levels. A healthier relationship with food, a deeper connection with the body's signals, and a reduction in the impact of stress on diabetes management are all benefits of mindfulness meditation. Mindful eating can become a lifelong habit that improves the lives of diabetics with support and consistent practice.

Techniques for Portion Control in Diabetes Management Portion control is an essential part of diabetes management. Diabetes patients can better control their blood sugar levels and keep a healthy weight by controlling how much food they eat at each meal. Techniques for portion control offer practical ways to control portion sizes, make better food choices, and control diabetes in general. The following are some efficient methods that can assist diabetics in maintaining a healthy weight and optimizing their diabetes management.

Utilize Measuring Tools: Utilizing estimating cups, spoons, and a kitchen scale can assist individuals with precisely estimating and control segment sizes. Estimating apparatuses give an objective method for deciding suitable serving sizes for various nutrition classes, like grains, proteins, and vegetables. A serving of cooked grains, for instance, should be about half a cup, and a serving of protein, such as chicken or fish, should be about the size of a deck of cards. Estimating devices can be especially useful in the early phases of part control, as they give a visual reference to legitimate piece sizes.

Establish visual cues: While eating out or in circumstances where estimating apparatuses may not be accessible, people can utilize obvious signs to appraise segment sizes. A serving of vegetables, for instance, should be about the size of a baseball, a serving of fruit should fit in your palm, and a serving of cheese should be about the size of two dice. These obvious signs can act as a supportive reference when confronted with new food segments.

Put non-starchy vegetables on half of your plate: Non-bland vegetables, like salad greens, broccoli, peppers, and zucchini, are low in calories and carbs while giving fundamental supplements and fiber. You can make a visually appealing meal while naturally reducing the space available for foods with more calories and carbohydrates by filling half of your plate with non-starchy vegetables. By emphasizing nutrient-dense, low-calorie options that support blood sugar management, this strategy encourages portion control.

Keep liquid calories in mind: It's easy to overlook the impact beverages have on portion control because they can significantly increase calorie and carbohydrate intake. Sugary drinks like soda, fruit juice, and coffee or tea sweetened with sugar can quickly raise blood sugar levels. Drinking water, herbal tea that hasn't been sweetened, or sugar-free alternatives can help you control your portion sizes and avoid overindulging in sugar. Because alcohol can also affect blood sugar control, it is essential to drink in moderation if you decide to do so.

Read labels on food: Serving sizes, calorie content, and carbohydrate counts can all be found by reading food labels. Individuals can better understand how much they are consuming and make informed decisions about portion control by paying attention to the portion sizes listed on food labels. Also, monitoring the starch content in food varieties is critical for people with diabetes, as carbs fundamentally affect glucose levels.

Practice the Plate Technique: A straightforward and efficient method for portion control is the plate method. It involves allocating specific portions to various food groups on your plate. Non-starchy vegetables should take up half of the plate, lean proteins should take up one quarter, and whole grains or starchy vegetables should take up the remaining quarter. This technique guarantees a reasonable feast that advances segment control and stable glucose levels.

Dial Back and Relish Your Dinners: Improving portion control can be helped by eating slowly and mindfully. When we eat slowly, we give our brains a chance to figure out when we've had enough because our bodies take time to feel full. Pay attention to your body's signals of hunger and fullness and chew each bite thoroughly. Mindful eating can help you eat less and control your portions more effectively.

Recognizing Hunger and Fullness Causes Diabetes management necessitates careful attention to nutrition and diet. Recognizing signals of hunger and fullness is an essential part of diabetes management. People with diabetes can better control their blood sugar levels and keep a healthy weight by understanding and responding to these cues. For effective diabetes management, this article examines the significance of recognizing hunger and fullness cues.

The body's way of telling you that it needs food is through hunger cues. However, due to fluctuations in blood sugar levels and the effects of certain medications, diabetics may experience alterations in their hunger cues. Diabetes patients must learn to recognize these cues and distinguish between genuine hunger and other sensations like cravings or emotional triggers.

Understanding the relationship between food intake and blood sugar levels is one important factor in recognizing hunger cues. At the point when glucose levels drop too low, the body triggers hunger signs to incite the admission of starches, which can rapidly raise glucose. Nevertheless, it is essential to exercise caution and select healthy carbohydrates over processed or sugary snacks. Entire grains, organic products, and vegetables are magnificent decisions as they give fundamental supplements and affect glucose levels.

The practice of portion control is another crucial aspect of recognizing hunger cues. By eating smaller, well-balanced meals and snacks at regular intervals throughout the day, diabetics frequently reap the benefits of this strategy. They can avoid extreme hunger and overeating by doing this. Individuals with diabetes can better manage their condition and avoid spikes in blood sugar by understanding portion sizes and following meal planning guidelines.

Then again, perceiving totality signs is similarly significant for diabetes control. In order to maintain stable blood sugar levels and manage weight, it is essential to eat until you are comfortably full rather than overeating. It requires investment for the cerebrum to enlist sensations of completion, so people ought to eat gradually and carefully, focusing on the body's signs.

To perceive completion signs successfully, killing interruptions during meals is significant. Mindless eating and excessive consumption can result from eating while working or watching television. Instead, people ought to concentrate on the food they're consuming, savoring each bite and paying attention to the flavors, textures, and sense of satisfaction it provides.

It's also a good idea to practice being aware of your portions. Utilizing more modest plates, bowls, and utensils can make the deception of a more significant piece, causing people to feel happy with less food. Additionally, since the body takes time to indicate that it is full, it is best to wait a few minutes before considering a second serving.

Emotional cues associated with eating are also essential for diabetes management. Numerous people with diabetes might go to nourishment for solace or as a survival strategy. Stress, fatigue,

misery, and different feelings can set off a craving to eat in any event, when not truly eager. Individuals can better manage their diabetes and avoid consuming excessive calories by becoming aware of these emotional cues and locating alternative means of addressing these feelings, such as engaging in physical activity or practicing relaxation techniques.

Another crucial aspect of diabetes management is regular exercise. Exercise can assist in weight management, improve insulin sensitivity, and regulate blood sugar levels. To ensure that the body is adequately fueled prior to and replenished after exercise, it is essential to recognize hunger and fullness cues. Consuming a reasonable feast or bite prior to practicing can give the essential energy, and perceiving completion prompts post-exercise can forestall gorging.

In conclusion, controlling diabetes requires understanding the signals of hunger and fullness. Individuals are able to make well-informed choices regarding their food choices and portion sizes if they are able to distinguish between genuine hunger and other sensations. Careful eating, segment control, and dealing with close to home signs connected with eating are fundamental systems for viable diabetes the executives.

METHODS FOR FEASTING OUT AND OVERSEEING SOCIAL CIRCUMSTANCES

Feasting out and exploring social circumstances can be trying for people with diabetes. The wealth of enticing food decisions, new menus, and companion strain can make it challenging to keep a solid eating routine and oversee glucose levels. Nonetheless, with appropriate preparation and a few supportive methodologies, people with diabetes can effectively explore these circumstances while getting a charge out of get-togethers. Dining out and managing social situations for diabetics are both covered in this article.

Make a plan:

If the restaurant's menu is online, look it up before you go. Search for better choices that line up with your dietary necessities. Numerous cafés now offer nourishment data on their sites, which can assist you with pursuing informed decisions. Choose a restaurant that serves a wide range of options, such as vegetables, whole grains, and lean proteins, if at all possible.

Share your dietary requirements:

Inform the waiter or waitress of your dietary restrictions and request any necessary adjustments. Most cafés are obliging and able to make acclimations to oblige extraordinary dietary requirements. You can control how much you consume by asking for sauces, dressings, and condiments to be served on the side.

Practice segment control: Frequently, restaurant portions are larger than necessary. When the meal is served, you should think about splitting a dish with a friend or asking for a to-go box, and portion out the appropriate amount before you start eating. You'll be able to better control your blood sugar levels and avoid overeating in this way.

Consider hidden sugars:

Focus on secret sugars in sauces, marinades, and dressings, as they can altogether affect glucose levels. Instead of frying, choose dishes that are grilled, baked, or steamed. You can control how much you eat by choosing low-sugar dressings or sauces or asking for them on the side.

Pick better cooking strategies: Prioritize dishes that are cooked in healthier ways, like grilling, steaming, or broiling, when choosing your meal. You'll be able to better control your blood sugar levels and reduce your intake of unhealthy fats thanks to these strategies.

Keep hydrated:

Choose your beverages with care. Sugary sodas, sweetened beverages, and alcoholic beverages are all bad for you because they are high in calories and can spike blood sugar. Choose sparkling water with a splash of citrus for flavor, unsweetened tea, or water.

Not just the food, but the company as well: Change your focus from food to socializing and having fun with other people. Instead of concentrating solely on the food, engage in conversation, take part in activities, and enjoy the moment. Changing one's perspective can help cut down on the urge to eat too much or choose unhealthy foods.

Prepare for pressure from others:

In social settings, you might feel pressured to eat unhealthy foods or eat more than you need. Set yourself up intellectually to pleasantly decline such offers or find options that line up with your dietary requirements. Keep in mind that you should put your health and well-being first.

Bring a nutritious dish: Assuming that you're going to a potluck or a get-together where you can add to the dinner, consider bringing a solid dish that you can appreciate irreproachable. You'll have at least one choice that meets your dietary needs this way.

Snacks for an emergency:

If you're in a situation where you need to quickly stabilize your blood sugar levels or there aren't many options, always carry emergency snacks like nuts, seeds, or a piece of fruit.

Keep moving: Integrate active work into your day, particularly previously or after a get-together. Walking or doing light exercise can help you control your blood sugar and improve your overall health.

Screen your glucose levels: It's critical to keep an eye on your blood sugar levels on a regular basis, especially after meals.

CHAPTER SIX
EXERCISE AND PHYSICAL ACTIVITY

Regular physical activity and exercise are essential for diabetes management and control. Physical activity not only aids diabetics in maintaining a healthy weight but also enhances insulin sensitivity, lowers blood sugar levels, and lowers the risk of diabetes complications. This article discusses the significance of physical activity and exercise in diabetes management and offers helpful suggestions for incorporating them into a diabetes management plan.

Benefits of Exercise to Control Diabetes: Diabetes patients can reap numerous benefits from exercise. It further develops insulin responsiveness, which permits the body to utilize insulin all the more really and keep up with stable glucose levels. Customary active work likewise advances weight the executives by consuming calories and building fit bulk. Additionally, exercise has been shown to reduce stress, improve cardiovascular health, lower blood pressure, and improve well-being in general.

EXERCISE OPTIONS:

There are different sorts of activity that people with diabetes can take part in to control their condition:

Physical Activity:

Heart rate and breathing are increased during aerobic activities like brisk walking, jogging, cycling, swimming, dancing, and aerobic classes. Aim for a minimum of 150 minutes of daily, moderate-intensity aerobic exercise.

Strength Workouts:

Using weights, resistance bands, or your own bodyweight, you can do strength training exercises that help build muscle strength and improve your overall body composition. Incorporate strength preparing practices a few times each week, focusing on significant muscle gatherings.

Balance And Flexibility Exercises:

Stretching and yoga, two forms of flexibility training, both increase range of motion and reduce the risk of injury. Yoga and tai chi are examples of balance exercises that can improve stability and lower the risk of falling.

Speak With A Medical Professional:

Prior to beginning an activity program, it's urgent to talk with a medical care proficient, like a specialist or a guaranteed diabetes instructor. They can help you make a customized exercise plan and offer advice on the kinds of exercises and intensity levels that are best for you.

Glucose Checking:

Consistently screen glucose levels previously, during, and after work out, particularly in the event that utilizing insulin or certain meds that can bring down glucose. This will enable any necessary adjustments to medication or food intake and help keep blood sugar levels within the acceptable range.

Begin Gradually And Progress Steadily:

If you are just getting started with exercise, start with low-impact activities and gradually increase the duration and intensity over time. The body is able to adapt to this method, which also lowers the likelihood of injuries. Don't push yourself past your limits; instead, listen to your body.

Keep Hydrated:

Drink a lot of water previously, during, and after exercise to remain hydrated. Blood sugar levels and overall performance can be impacted by dehydration. During your workout, keep a water bottle nearby and drink frequently.

Wear the Right Shoes: Pick agreeable, well-fitting athletic shoes that offer sufficient help and padding. Foot problems and injuries can be avoided with the right footwear, which is especially important for diabetics.

Take Safety Measures into Account:

Use appropriate safety gear and wear reflective clothing when participating in outdoor activities like cycling or walking. Additionally, it is advisable to carry diabetes-related identification and emergency contact information.

Stir Up Your Everyday practice:

To maintain motivation and avoid boredom, variety is essential. Include a variety of exercises into your routine to keep your workouts enjoyable and target various muscle groups.

Throughout the day, be active:

Recollect that actual work isn't restricted to organized practice meetings. If you work a sedentary job, find ways to get more movement into your day by taking the stairs instead of the elevator, parking farther from where you want to go, or taking short breaks to stretch and walk around.

THE JOB OF PRACTICE IN DIABETES CONTROL

Practice assumes a critical part in the administration and control of diabetes. For diabetics, engaging in regular physical activity has a number of advantages that can have a significant impact on blood sugar levels, insulin sensitivity, weight management, and overall health. This article investigates the significance of practice in diabetes control and gives important bits of knowledge into how exercise can be integrated into a diabetes the executives plan.

Further Developed Insulin Awareness:

Practice further develops insulin responsiveness, permitting the body to successfully utilize insulin more. Muscles require glucose for energy while exercising. As a result, muscles absorb more glucose, which aids in lowering blood sugar levels. Customary activity can improve insulin responsiveness, making it simpler for the body to keep up with stable glucose levels.

Glucose Guideline:

Participating in active work directs glucose levels in different ways. Practice animates the take-up of glucose by muscles, decreasing how much glucose flowing in the circulatory system. It likewise advances the vehicle of glucose into cells freely of insulin, which is especially useful for people with type 2 diabetes or insulin obstruction. Additionally, even after an activity has been completed, it may continue to lower blood sugar levels.

Weight The Executives:

In order to control diabetes, it is essential to maintain a healthy weight because excess weight can exacerbate insulin resistance and cause complications. By increasing metabolism and burning calories, exercise aids in weight management. It likewise assists work with inclining bulk, which adds to a higher metabolic rate. For diabetics, engaging in regular physical activity and eating a well-balanced diet can aid in weight loss and maintenance.

Health Of The Heart:

Diabetes raises the risk of cardiovascular problems like stroke and heart disease. Practice assumes a critical part in working on cardiovascular wellbeing by diminishing pulse, further developing blood dissemination, and bringing down LDL (terrible) cholesterol levels. Cardiovascular disease risk can be reduced through regular aerobic exercise, such as swimming, brisk walking, jogging, cycling, and swimming.

Stress Decrease:

The management of diabetes as a whole and blood sugar levels can be negatively impacted by stress. Because it encourages the production of endorphins—also known as "feel-good" hormones—which have the ability to improve mood and alleviate stress—exercise is an effective method for reducing stress. Taking part in actual work, whether it's an exercise at the rec center, a nature walk, or a yoga class, can give a psychological and close to home lift, assisting individuals with better adapting to the difficulties of overseeing diabetes.

Further Developed Pulse And Blood Lipid Profile:

It has been demonstrated that exercise can lower blood pressure and improve blood lipid profile, lowering the risk of hypertension and other cardiovascular complications. The heart is strengthened, blood flow is improved, HDL (good) cholesterol levels are raised, and triglycerides and LDL (bad) cholesterol levels are reduced when people exercise regularly. These enhancements add to better by and large cardiovascular wellbeing in people with diabetes.

Upgraded Nature Of Rest:

Sleep patterns can be disrupted by diabetes, which can result in insomnia or poor quality sleep. Exercise can decidedly influence rest by advancing a more tranquil and more profound rest. However, intense exercise close to bedtime should be avoided because it may make it difficult to fall asleep and increase alertness. Finishing exercise meetings essentially a couple of hours before bedtime is ideal.

A Greater Level Of Energy:

Diabetes patients can combat feelings of fatigue and increase their energy levels through regular exercise. Exercise boosts overall stamina, increases oxygen and nutrient delivery to the muscles, and improves the efficiency of the cardiovascular and respiratory systems. Consequently, increased energy and vitality are frequently cited as a direct result of exercise.

Prevention of complications from diabetes: Diabetes-related complications, such as cardiovascular disease, nerve damage, kidney disease, and eye issues, can all be reduced with exercise. by controlling weight, improving overall health, and maintaining healthy blood sugar levels.

CHOOSING THE PERFECT EXERCISE ROUTINE

For achieving your fitness objectives and maintaining a healthy lifestyle, selecting the appropriate exercise routine is crucial. There is no one-size-fits-all approach to exercising. Preferences, fitness levels, and health considerations vary greatly among individuals. By understanding your requirements and inclinations, you can pick a work-out schedule that is agreeable, supportable, and successful. You can use the helpful advice in this article to choose the best exercise routine for you.

Check Your Objectives: Begin by deciding your wellness objectives. Are you trying to reduce stress, build strength, lose weight, increase flexibility, or improve your cardiovascular health? Choosing exercises that are in line with your objectives will be easier if you know what your objectives are.

Think About Your Interests: It doesn't have to be a chore to exercise. Think about activities that you truly enjoy. Walking, jogging, hiking, cycling, and other outdoor activities might be your thing. Group fitness classes or team sports might be more engaging for you if you prefer to be in a group setting. If you choose activities that you enjoy, you are more likely to stick to your exercise plan.

Assess Your Wellness Level: Take a genuine evaluation of your ongoing wellness level. Start with low-impact activities if you're new to exercise or haven't been active in a while and gradually increase the intensity and duration over time. Consult a doctor or other medical professional before beginning any exercise program if you have any existing health conditions.

Think About Your Schedule: Take a look at your schedule and figure out how much time you can exercise realistically. Pick exercises that can be effortlessly integrated into your day to day daily schedule. Even short workouts, like 10-minute walks throughout the day, can have a positive impact on one's health. Look for workouts that save you time, like high-intensity interval training (HIIT), which combines short bursts of intense exercise with periods of rest, if you have a busy schedule.

Assortment and Equilibrium: Try to incorporate a variety of cardiovascular, strength, and flexibility exercises into your daily routine. Cardiovascular activities, like strolling, running, swimming, or moving, further develop heart wellbeing and consume calories. Using weights or resistance bands, you can do strength training exercises that help you burn more calories and build lean muscle mass. Yoga and other flexibility exercises like stretching can increase range of motion and prevent injuries. In order to target various muscle groups and maintain overall fitness, try to keep your workouts balanced.

Seek Advice from a Professional: Consider seeking guidance from a certified fitness professional or personal trainer if you are unsure of where to begin or how to perform particular exercises. They can help you figure out how fit you are, give you specific workout suggestions, and show you how to avoid injuries by using proper form and technique.

Take Note of Your Body: Pay attention to how different exercises affect your body. Alter or select a different exercise that is better suited to your body if an activity causes pain or discomfort. When starting a new routine, it's important to challenge yourself but also to know your limits and not push yourself too hard.

Continuous Movement: Over time, gradually increase the

difficulty, duration, and intensity of your exercises. Your body will be able to adapt to this method, which also lowers the likelihood of overuse injuries. Beginning with shorter workouts, gradually increase the duration as your fitness level rises. In a similar vein, gradually increase the intensity of your workouts to test your body without putting too much stress on it.

Make it a Social Movement: Practicing with a companion, relative, or joining bunch wellness classes can make your exercises more pleasant and propelling. Having a workout buddy can help you stay on track, encourage you, and make exercising feel less lonely.

Observe and adjust: Consistently screen your advancement and reconsider your work-out daily schedule.

Tips For Including Physical Activity in Your Daily Routine Managing and controlling diabetes necessitates including physical activity in your daily routine. Improved insulin sensitivity, better control of blood sugar levels, better weight management, and a lower risk of diabetes complications are all benefits of regular exercise. However, it can be difficult to fit physical activity into a busy schedule. This article gives important hints to integrating actual work into your everyday existence for powerful diabetes control.

Set attainable goals: Begin by setting physical activity goals that are attainable and attainable. Aim for a minimum of 150 minutes of daily, moderate-intensity aerobic exercise. Break it down into manageable chunks, like exercising for 30 minutes five days a week or three sessions of 10 minutes each day. Laying out feasible objectives improves the probability of achievement and assists you with remaining propelled.

Identify Opportunities For Activities: Throughout the day, look for opportunities to get active. If possible, walk or bike to work, take the stairs rather than the elevator, or park further away from your destination to get more steps in. Track down ways of integrating active work into your day to day daily practice, like planting, family tasks, or strolling the canine. Each and every piece of development adds up and adds to your general movement level.

It should be a priority: Include physical activity as a priority in your daily schedule. Treat it as a significant arrangement that you can't miss. Set a particular time for work out, whether it's toward the beginning of the day, during mid-day break, or at night, and stick to it. Consistency is critical to laying out a propensity and making actual work an ordinary piece of your life.

Find Exercises You Appreciate: To make physical activity more enjoyable and long-lasting, choose activities that you truly enjoy. Find something that makes you happy, whether it's dancing, swimming, hiking, playing a sport, or taking a fitness class. You are more likely to look forward to the activity and keep doing it over time if you enjoy it.

Socialize it: Participate in group exercise classes or engage in physical activity with friends, family, or colleagues. Having an exercise pal or partaking in bunch exercises makes practice more pleasant as well as gives responsibility and backing. Together, you can inspire and test one another, making the experience more enjoyable and rewarding.

Divide it up into smaller steps: Break exercise down into smaller sessions if it seems hard to find uninterrupted time. Short episodes of active work over the course of the day can be similarly as viable. Take a brisk walk during your lunch break, for instance, or perform a quick home workout in the morning and evening. Even if you do physical activity in smaller amounts, it still has a big impact on your health.

Make television Time Dynamic: Rather than sitting on the lounge chair while staring at the television, utilize that opportunity to take part in light actual work. Use an exercise bike or treadmill, do stretches or exercises during commercial breaks, or do simple household chores like dusting or folding laundry while watching your favorite shows. Along these lines, you can integrate actual work into your recreation time.

Investigate Technology: Make physical activity more fun by utilizing technology. Set goals, track your progress, and track your steps with fitness apps or wearable devices. Numerous applications offer exercise routine schedules, directed works out, and persuasive elements to keep you on target. You can likewise attempt online exercise recordings or virtual wellness classes that give adaptability and assortment.

Include Everyone In The Family: Include family time with physical activity. Plan open air exercises or games that get everybody rolling, like climbing, cycling, or playing sports. This not only encourages you to exercise, but it also encourages your family members to live healthy, active lives.

MANAGING BLOOD SUGAR LEVELS DURING EXERCISE

Exercise is an essential part of diabetes management because it helps regulate blood sugar levels, improve insulin sensitivity, and improve overall health. However, in order to avoid hypoglycemia (low blood sugar) or hyperglycemia (high blood sugar), diabetics must monitor their blood sugar levels while exercising. For effective diabetes management, this article provides useful tips for controlling blood sugar levels while exercising.

Screen Glucose Levels:

Keeping an eye on your blood sugar levels before, during, and after exercise is absolutely necessary. Customary observing assists you with understanding how your body answers various sorts and powers of actual work. Before beginning your workout, check your blood sugar levels to make sure they are within the recommended range. If your blood sugar is too low (below 100 mg/dL, or 5.6 mmol/L) or too high, (above 250 mg/dL, or 13.9 mmol/L), you may need to modify your exercise routine.

Modify Insulin And Medication:

Your diabetes medication or insulin dose may need to be adjusted based on your blood sugar levels and the type of exercise you are doing. Determine the most effective method for managing your insulin or medication regimen while exercising with your healthcare team. They can give direction on timing, measurements changes, and any fundamental insurances to keep away from hypoglycemia or hyperglycemia.

When To Exercise: Think about when you exercise and when you eat and get insulin injections. To reduce the risk of hypoglycemia, it is generally advised to refrain from exercising during insulin's peak activity. If you take insulin before eating, plan your workouts at least two to three hours after eating or inject insulin into a muscle group that doesn't need it.

Consumption of Carbohydrates: To keep your blood sugar levels stable, you may need to consume carbohydrates, but this will depend on how long you exercise and how hard you work. Prevent hypoglycemia by having a small snack before or during longer or more strenuous workouts or by eating fast-acting carbohydrates like fruit juice, glucose tablets, or sports drinks. Find the amount and source of carbohydrates that work best for you by experimenting.

Hydration:

To support optimal blood sugar regulation during exercise, it is essential to drink enough water. To stay hydrated before, during, and after your workout, drink plenty of water. A lack of water can raise blood sugar levels. However, avoid sugary drinks because they may spike blood sugar. When you can, go with water or sugar-free options.

Warm-Up And Cool-Down In Stages:

Your exercise routine should include a gradual warm-up and cool-down period. This prevents rapid changes in blood sugar levels and helps your body get ready for physical activity. Begin with 5-10 minutes of low-power work out, like strolling or extending, prior to advancing to additional lively exercises. Moreover, finish your exercise with a couple of moments of delicate development and extending to progressively bring your pulse and glucose levels back to typical.

Pick The Right Force:

The power of your activity can essentially influence glucose levels. For diabetics, moderate-intensity aerobic activities like cycling or brisk walking are generally recommended. When you exercise at a high intensity, especially if you take insulin or other medications for diabetes, your blood sugar levels may drop quickly. Determine the appropriate exercise intensity for your condition by consulting your healthcare team.

Prepare for the unexpected: During exercise, you should always carry glucose gels or tablets, which are sources of fast-acting carbohydrates. These can be utilized to rapidly raise your glucose levels in the event that you experience hypoglycemia side effects, like discombobulation, disarray, or perspiring .

CHAPTER SEVEN
MANAGING STRESS AND GETTING ENOUGH SLEEP

Stress management and sleep are important for managing diabetes and overall health. Blood sugar levels, insulin resistance, and the capacity to effectively manage diabetes can all be directly impacted by stress. Moreover, lacking or low quality rest can disturb glucose guideline and add to different unexpected problems. This article examines the significance of managing stress and getting enough sleep for diabetes management and offers useful methods for enhancing well-being in these areas.

Stress Reduction:

Recognize the Sources of Stress: Find out what factors increase your stress levels. This might incorporate business related pressures, monetary worries, relationship issues, or everyday problems. Perceiving your pressure triggers can assist you with creating powerful survival methods.

Practice Unwinding Methods:

Relaxation techniques can help you deal with stress. Yoga, deep breathing exercises, meditation, mindfulness, and other forms of yoga can help you relax and feel less stressed. Integrate these practices into your everyday daily schedule, especially during seasons of increased pressure.

Regular Sport:

Not only is exercise good for managing diabetes, but it also helps reduce stress. Taking part in normal activity helps discharge endorphins, which are regular temperament sponsors. Pick exercises you appreciate and go for the gold 30 minutes of moderate-power practice most days of the week.

Using Time Productively:

Stress can be made worse by not managing your time well. Make tasks a priority, establish attainable objectives, and divide larger projects into smaller, more manageable tasks. Learning how to effectively manage your time can help you feel more in control and reduce stress.

Seek Assistance:

Share your feelings and concerns with family, friends, or support groups. Emotional support, practical advice, and a sense of connection can all come from having a support network. Proficient guiding or treatment can likewise be gainful in overseeing pressure.

Solid Way Of Life:

Stress can be reduced by leading a healthy lifestyle. Maintain a healthy diet, engage in regular exercise, limit alcohol consumption, and avoid smoking. These lifestyle choices can help lower stress levels and support overall well-being.

SLEEP HYGIENE:

Create a routine:

By going to bed and getting up at the same time each day, even on weekends, you can establish a routine for getting enough sleep. Better sleep quality and internal clock regulation are both aided by this routine.

Create An Environment That Encourages Sleep:

Make your room helpful for rest. Keep the room quiet, cool, and dark. White noise machines, earplugs, or eye masks may be used to block out distracting light and sounds.

Beware Of Stimulants:

Caffeine and nicotine can disrupt sleep, so do not consume them close to bedtime. Additionally, to avoid discomfort and nighttime awakenings, avoid large meals, spicy foods, and excessive fluids before bed.

Relax Before Going To Bed:

Before going to bed, start a relaxing routine to let your body know it's time to sleep. Read, take a warm bath, listen to soothing music, or practice relaxation techniques are all calming activities.

Keep Away From Electronic Gadgets:

Electronic devices' blue light can make it hard to sleep. Avoid using computers, smartphones, or tablets for at least an hour before going to bed. To reduce the impact on the quality of your sleep, think about using devices with nighttime modes or blue light filters.

Reduce Stress:

Sleep quality can be significantly impacted by stress. Before going to bed, try stress management techniques like deep breathing, meditation, or journaling to help you relax.

Regular Sport:

Quality of sleep can be improved by doing regular physical activity during the day. However, avoid vigorous exercise close to bedtime because it may make it harder to fall asleep and increase alertness. Try to finish your workouts at least a few hours before you go to bed.

Assess Medication:

A few meds can disturb rest designs. Assuming you suspect that your diabetes meds or different drugs are influencing your rest, examine this with your family specialist.

THE IMPACT OF STRESS ON BLOOD SUGAR LEVELS

Although stress is a natural part of life, it can significantly affect many aspects of our health, including blood sugar levels. Stress management is especially important for diabetics because it can have a direct impact on blood glucose control and diabetes management as a whole. Diabetes management requires an understanding of the relationship between stress and blood sugar levels. This article looks at how stress affects blood sugar levels and offers ways to manage stress to control diabetes better.

Stress Reaction and Glucose Levels: Our bodies produce stress hormones like cortisol and adrenaline when we are under stress. The "fight-or-flight" response is sparked by these hormones, which raise blood sugar, heart rate, and blood pressure. This physiological reaction is intended to give energy during an apparent danger or risk. This stress response has the potential to raise blood sugar levels in diabetics.

Stress and Insulin Obstruction: Constant pressure can add to insulin obstruction, a condition in which cells become less receptive with the impacts of insulin. At the point when insulin obstruction happens, glucose can't enter the cells really, prompting raised glucose levels. High levels of stress hormones can make it harder for insulin to control blood sugar, which could make it harder to control diabetes.

When stressed, a lot of people turn to food for comfort, which leads to emotional eating. Stress-related close to home eating frequently includes devouring fatty, sweet, or unfortunate food sources, which can cause glucose levels to spike. Moreover, close to home eating can add to weight gain and trouble overseeing diabetes really.

Coping Mechanisms And Habits Of Life: Stress can also have an effect on our coping mechanisms and habits of life, which can make it harder to control blood sugar. Some people may use unhealthy coping mechanisms like smoking, drinking too much alcohol, or not taking care of their diabetes. These actions have the potential to alter blood sugar levels and contribute to health problems in the long run.

STRATEGIES FOR MANAGING STRESS AND CONTROLLING BLOOD SUGAR:

Distinguish Pressure Triggers:

Identify the events, situations, or circumstances in your life that cause stress. You can take proactive measures to manage or avoid these triggers whenever possible by identifying them. The first step in developing effective strategies for managing stress is awareness.

Stress Decrease Methods:

Include strategies for reducing stress in your daily routine. Take part in activities that help you relax, like yoga, tai chi, deep breathing exercises, or meditation. These practices can assist with bringing down pressure chemicals, lessen uneasiness, and advance better glucose control.

Customary Active Work:

Physical activity helps control diabetes and is an effective stress management strategy. Regular exercise helps lower blood sugar levels, improve mood, and reduce stress. Go for the gold 150 minutes of moderate-power high-impact practice each week, like energetic strolling, swimming, or cycling.

Support Structure:

Look for help from family, friends, or support groups. When you talk about your worries and experiences with other people who can relate, you can get emotional support and reduce stress. If you need help, you might want to join a diabetes support group or get professional counseling.

Using Time Productively:

Stress levels can be exacerbated by inadequate time management. Set attainable objectives, prioritize tasks, and divide larger projects into manageable steps. Learning how to effectively manage your time can help you feel more in control and reduce stress.

Choices For A Healthy Lifestyle:

A healthy lifestyle can aid in stress reduction and improve blood sugar control. Eat a well-balanced diet that is full of fruits and vegetables, lean proteins, and whole grains. Reduce your intake of processed and sugary foods. Stress management and blood sugar regulation can also be helped by getting enough sleep, practicing good sleep hygiene, and avoiding too much alcohol and caffeine.

Methods Of Relaxation:

Find the best relaxation method for you by experimenting with a variety of methods. This could involve journaling, guided imagery, progressive muscle relaxation, deep breathing exercises, or both.

TECHNIQUES FOR REDUCING STRESS AND RELAXING

In the fast-paced world of today, stress has become an everyday occurrence. Managing stress is important for our overall health and can improve our mental and physical health as well as other aspects of our health. This article looks at different ways to relax and reduce stress that can help you manage stress better and bring calm and balance to your life.

Exercises In Deep Breathing:

Deep breathing is a simple but effective method for promoting relaxation and stress reduction. Take slow, full breaths, breathing in through your nose and breathing out through your mouth. Center around the impression of your breath as it enters and leaves your body. Anxiety can be reduced, heart rate can be slowed, and your nervous system can be calmed with deep breathing.

PMR, Or Progressive Muscle Relaxation,:

PMR includes straining and afterward delivering different muscle gatherings to advance unwinding. Start by tensing the muscles in one part of your body, like your hands, for a few seconds. Then, focus on the feeling of relaxation while you let go of the tension. Move methodicallly through your body, straining and delivering each muscle bunch. Relaxation and muscle tension relief are both aided by this method.

Meditation On Mindfulness:

Care reflection includes focusing on the current second without judgment. Track down a peaceful and agreeable space, and concentrate on your breath, substantial sensations, or a particular item. At the point when your psyche meanders, delicately take it back to the current second. Mindfulness meditation can help you feel less stressed out, become more aware of yourself, and feel better all around.

Yoga:

Yoga helps people relax and feel less stressed by incorporating meditation, controlled breathing, and physical postures. Regular yoga practice has been shown to improve flexibility, strength, and balance, as well as to calm the mind and alleviate anxiety. Learn various yoga poses and sequences that are appropriate for your fitness level by enrolling in a class or by utilizing online resources.

Directed Symbolism:

Utilizing your imagination to create a mental image that encourages calm and relaxation is guided imagery. Close your eyes and imagine yourself in a peaceful and serene setting, such as a beach or a forest, in a quiet and comfortable location. Visualize the sights, sounds, and smells of that environment to engage your senses. This strategy can assist with moving your concentrate away from stressors and instigate a condition of unwinding.**Journaling:**

Writing down your feelings, worries, and thoughts can help you feel better and relieve stress. Put away a couple of moments every day to diary about your encounters, feelings, and any stressors you're confronting. Gaining perspective, recognizing patterns, and releasing negative emotions are all benefits of this practice. You can also use journaling to focus on the good things in your life and express gratitude.

Taking Part In Leisure Activities:

Participating in activities you enjoy can help you relax and reduce stress. Commit time to side interests or exercises that give you pleasure, whether it's painting, planting, playing an instrument, or moving. By participating in these activities, you can focus on the present, experience flow, and detach from stressors.

Social Assistance:

For stress reduction, it is essential to seek social support and connect with loved ones. Talk about your thoughts and worries with confided in companions or relatives. Spend time together, talk about important things, and look for comfort in their support. A sense of connection and belonging can also be gained by participating in community activities or joining support groups.

Perform Physical Activity:

Not only is regular exercise good for your health, but it also helps you feel better and less stressed out. Take part in activities you enjoy, like cycling, walking, running, dancing, or Go for the gold 30 minutes of moderate-power practice most days of the week.

The importance of good sleep in diabetes management Sleep is important to our overall health and well-being. Our bodies go through crucial processes for healing, restoration, and metabolic regulation while we sleep. Quality sleep is especially important for diabetics because it has a direct impact on blood sugar control and diabetes management as a whole. This article examines the significance of good sleep in diabetes management and offers suggestions for enhancing sleep routines for better diabetes management.

Consequences For Insulin Sensitivity: Quality rest is firmly connected to insulin responsiveness. At the point when we rest, our bodies direct the creation and arrival of different chemicals, including insulin. Insulin resistance, a condition in which the body's cells become less responsive to insulin, can be caused by insufficient or poor sleep. As a result, glucose is unable to enter the cells efficiently, resulting in elevated blood sugar levels. It is possible to improve insulin sensitivity and maintain better blood sugar control by improving sleep quality.

Control Of Glucose: Sleep quality is important for keeping blood sugar levels stable throughout the day. Hormonal imbalances that affect glucose regulation can be caused by insufficient sleep or irregular sleep patterns. It can prompt expanded glucose levels, higher HbA1c levels (a proportion of long haul glucose control), and a more serious gamble of creating type 2 diabetes. Getting enough and uninterrupted sleep on a regular basis can help maintain stable glycemic control and lower the risk of diabetes complications.

Hunger and Food Admission: Sleep deprivation can change the hormones that control appetite, making you feel hungry and want to eat more, especially foods that are high in calories and carbohydrates. Maintaining a healthy diet and effectively controlling blood sugar levels may be difficult due to this. Good sleep helps regulate appetite hormones like leptin and ghrelin, which in turn aids in maintaining a healthy diet and managing diabetes.

Activity Levels and Energy Levels: It is essential to get a good night's sleep in order to support physical activity and replenish energy levels. It can be more difficult to maintain a regular exercise routine, which is essential for managing diabetes, when you don't get enough sleep because it can cause fatigue, decreased motivation, and decreased physical performance. You can ensure that you have the energy and drive to engage in physical activity and maintain an active lifestyle by making quality sleep a priority.

Stress and Profound Prosperity: Sleep quality has a significant impact on emotional well-being and stress levels. Absence of rest can increment stress chemical levels, prompting increased tension, peevishness, and emotional episodes. Stress and close to home unsettling influences can influence glucose control and make it more testing to successfully oversee diabetes. You can improve your emotional well-being, reduce stress levels, and create a more conducive environment for diabetes management by placing a high value on quality sleep.

TIPS FOR GETTING A BETTER NIGHT'S SLEEP:

Establish A Regular Sleep Routine:

Set an ordinary rest plan by hitting the hay and awakening simultaneously consistently, including ends of the week. This manages your body's interior clock and advances better rest quality.

Make Your Space Sleep-Friendly:

Make your bedroom a place where you can sleep in comfort. Guarantee your sleeping pad, cushions, and bedding are agreeable and strong. Keep the room quiet, cool, and dark. White noise machines, earplugs, or eye masks may be used to block out distracting light and sounds.

Beware Of Stimulants:

Caffeine and nicotine, two stimulants that can disrupt sleep, should not be consumed close to bedtime. Additionally, to avoid discomfort and nighttime awakenings, avoid large meals, spicy foods, and excessive fluids before bed.

Create A Bedtime Schedule:

To signal to your body that it is time to wind down and get ready for sleep, create a relaxing routine before bed. Take part in activities like reading, relaxing in a warm bath, learning how to relax, or listening to soothing music.

Establishing healthy sleeping habits is important for our overall health and well-being. It is essential for sustaining optimal daytime performance, supporting cognitive function, and promoting mental and physical rejuvenation. Be that as it may, numerous people battle with rest related issues, which can altogether affect their personal satisfaction. Laying out solid rest propensities is vital to further developing rest quality and guaranteeing serene evenings. In this article, we will look at practical strategies and tips for getting a good night's sleep.

Maintain A Regular Sleep Schedule: Keeping a consistent sleep schedule is one of the most important factors in improving the quality of your sleep. Even on weekends, try to get to bed and get up at the same time every day. Your body's internal clock is regulated by this regularity, making it simpler to naturally fall asleep and wake up. For establishing a healthy sleep-wake cycle, consistency is essential.

Establish A Calming Routine For Bedtime: Your body may receive a signal that it is time to unwind and prepare for sleep if you establish a relaxing bedtime routine. Take part in activities that help you relax, like reading, taking a hot bath, or practicing meditation. Try not to animate exercises or openness to splendid screens, as the blue light transmitted by electronic gadgets can upset your rest designs.

Make Your Space Sleep-Friendly: The environment you sleep in has a big impact on how well you sleep. Guarantee that your room is cool, calm, and dull. Put resources into an agreeable sleeping pad, cushions, and bedding that offer satisfactory help for your body. Use power outage drapes or an eye cover to shut out any outside light sources. To block out distracting sounds, think about using white noise machines or earplugs.

Reduce Your Intake Of Stimulants: Caffeine, nicotine, and alcohol are stimulants that can make it hard to fall asleep and stay asleep. Try not to consume these substances, particularly at night hours. Be aware of hidden sources of caffeine, such as chocolate and certain medications. Instead, choose herbal tea or beverages devoid of caffeine.

Make Your Bedroom a Relaxing Space: Your bedroom ought to be primarily used for rest and sleep. Work, watch TV, or scroll through your phone should not be done in your bed. You can train your mind and body to prepare for restful nights when you enter your bedroom by associating it with sleep.

Regularly Engage in Physical Activity: Normal activity can essentially further develop rest quality. Participating in actual work lessens feelings of anxiety, advance unwinding, and manage your rest wake cycle. Go for the gold 30 minutes of moderate-power practice most days of the week. However, avoid engaging in strenuous exercise too close to bedtime because it may rouse you and make it harder to fall asleep.

Reduce Stress: Anxiety and stress can have a significant impact on your ability to fall and stay asleep. Include strategies for stress management into your daily routine, such as journaling, deep breathing exercises, and mindfulness meditation. Engaging in a hobby, spending time in nature, or listening to calming music are all good ways to unwind and relax.

Make your bedroom a comfortable place to sleep: Make sure your sleeping environment is comfortable and conducive to good sleep by paying attention to it. Set the temperature in your bedroom so that you can sleep comfortably. Pick breathable and agreeable sleepwear and bedding materials. Think about getting a pillow that keeps your neck and spine in the right position.

Stop Urinating: On the off chance that you experience difficulty nodding off around evening time, it very well might be useful to restrict daytime snoozing. If you do take a nap, limit it to no more than 20 to 30 minutes and do not nap too close to your intended bedtime. Snoozing for a really long time or late in the day can disrupt your rest wake cycle.

CHAPTER EIGHT

MONITORING AND TRACKING PROGRESS

Diabetes is a chronic condition that necessitates ongoing management and monitoring to ensure that blood sugar levels remain under optimal control. Understanding how your lifestyle choices, medications, and treatment plans affect your diabetes control necessitate regular monitoring and tracking of your progress. You can better manage your diabetes by keeping an eye on key indicators and your progress on a regular basis, recognizing patterns, and making necessary adjustments. In this article, we will talk about how important it is to monitor and track progress in managing diabetes and offer helpful advice on how to do so effectively.

Glucose Checking:

A crucial part of managing diabetes is having your blood sugar checked on a regular basis. It lets you see how well you control your blood sugar levels and make any necessary adjustments. Determine the target range for your blood sugar levels and the frequency of testing with your healthcare team. At home, measure your blood sugar levels with a blood glucose meter. During your checkups, share a record of your readings with your healthcare provider.

CGM, Or Continuous Glucose Monitoring,:

Throughout the day, CGM systems provide real-time data on your blood sugar levels. These gadgets utilize a sensor embedded under the skin to gauge glucose levels in the interstitial liquid. CGM systems can help you understand how your blood sugar changes as a result of eating, exercising, and other things. You may be able to identify patterns and make adjustments to your diabetes management plan by reviewing the data from your CGM.

A1C Testing:

Your average blood sugar levels over the past two to three months are measured by the A1C test. It gives a general image of your glucose control and is regularly used to evaluate long haul diabetes the board. The majority of diabetics should aim for an A1C level below 7%, according to the American Diabetes Association. The frequency of your A1C testing should be discussed with your healthcare provider, and you can use the results to monitor your progress over time.

Food and Action Following:

Understanding how your diet and physical activity affect your blood sugar levels can be improved by keeping a food and activity diary. Record the kinds of food varieties you devour, segment sizes, and any pertinent data, for example, sugar content. Essentially, track your actual work, including term and force. By following your food and movement, you can distinguish patterns, decide what certain food sources or exercises mean for your glucose levels, and make changes in like manner.

Insulin And Medication Monitoring:

Assuming you take medicine or insulin to deal with your diabetes, observing their adequacy and potential secondary effects is significant. Keep track of your medication doses and times, as well as any fasting or post-meal changes in your blood sugar levels. This information can assist you and your healthcare provider in determining whether medication regimen adjustments are required.

Standard Medical Services Check-Ups:

Your healthcare provider needs to see you on a regular basis to keep an eye on your diabetes management and your progress. Discuss your blood sugar levels, A1C results, medication use, and any issues or difficulties you are having during these appointments. Your healthcare provider can assess your progress, offer direction, and modify your treatment plan if necessary.

Use Diabetes The Board Applications And Innovation:

You can monitor and track various aspects of your diabetes control with the help of a variety of digital tools and apps for diabetes management. You can frequently keep track of your blood sugar levels, take medications, eat, exercise, and other activities with these apps. Some applications even give bits of knowledge, patterns, and suggestions to assist you with keeping focused with your diabetes the board objectives.

Celebrate accomplishments and set goals: Setting explicit, reachable objectives can be rousing and give a feeling of achievement as you gain ground in your diabetes control. Separate bigger objectives into more modest, noteworthy stages.

THE SIGNIFICANCE OF REGULAR BLOOD SUGAR LEVEL MONITORING

Regular blood sugar level monitoring is an essential component of diabetes management and optimal control. High blood sugar levels are a hallmark of diabetes, a long-term condition caused by either a lack of insulin production or an inability to use insulin properly. Diabetes patients can gain valuable insights into their condition, make informed decisions regarding their treatment plan, and take proactive measures to effectively manage their diabetes by monitoring their blood sugar levels on a regular basis. In this article, we will discuss the significance and advantages of regular blood sugar monitoring for diabetes management.

Understanding How People React To Food And Medicine:

Various factors, such as diet, physical activity, medication, stress, and illness, can have an impact on blood sugar levels. Diabetes patients can learn how various foods and medications affect their blood sugar levels with regular monitoring. By following their glucose readings when feasts, they can recognize examples and arrive at informed conclusions about food decisions and drug changes in accordance with keep up with stable glucose levels.

Hyperglycemia And Hypoglycemia Early Detection:

Both hypoglycemia (low blood sugar) and hyperglycemia (high

blood sugar) can be quickly detected and treated with regular monitoring. Hyperglycemia can prompt long haul confusions, for example, nerve harm, kidney illness, and cardiovascular issues. Then again, hypoglycemia can cause prompt side effects like discombobulation, disarray, and even loss of awareness. Individuals are able to recognize these fluctuations and take the necessary precautions to prevent complications by regularly monitoring their blood sugar levels.

Planned Treatment Modifications:

Diabetes the board frequently includes various treatment systems, including way of life alterations, medicine, and insulin treatment. For healthcare providers to evaluate the efficacy of the current treatment plan, regular blood sugar monitoring provides crucial data. In the event that glucose levels reliably fall outside the objective reach, changes can be made to the treatment routine, for example, adjusting drug measurements or timing, investigating elective prescriptions, or taking into account insulin treatment. Based on each patient's unique blood sugar patterns, monitoring makes it possible to develop individualized treatment plans.

Following Long Haul Diabetes Control:

An indication of long-term blood sugar control is the measurement of glycosylated hemoglobin (HbA1c). HbA1c mirrors the typical glucose levels over the beyond a few months. Individuals and healthcare providers can monitor the effectiveness of diabetes management over time with regular HbA1c monitoring. In order to achieve better control and lower the risk of complications, consistently elevated HbA1c levels may indicate the need for treatment modifications or lifestyle adjustments.

Increasing Your Power And Self-Management:

Standard glucose observing enables people with diabetes to partake in their own consideration effectively. It helps them comprehend how their lifestyle choices affect their blood sugar levels and gives them real-time information about their condition. People are able to control their diabetes management and make decisions based on this information. It improves self-management and overall well-being by fostering a sense of empowerment, self-awareness, and responsibility.

Identifying Problem Areas And Patterns:

Keeping tabs on one's blood sugar levels makes it easier to spot patterns and trouble spots in one's control of diabetes. For instance, after consuming certain foods or beverages, some people may notice that their blood sugar levels consistently rise. They can make informed dietary choices to reduce fluctuations in blood sugar by recognizing these patterns. Likewise, following glucose levels when active work can assist people with deciding the proper timing and power of activity to keep up with stable glucose levels.

Enhancing Well-Being:

Through regular blood sugar monitoring, effective diabetes management can significantly enhance a person's quality of life. By keeping glucose levels inside target goes, the gamble of diabetes-related complexities can be decreased.

The management of diabetes necessitates careful attention to a variety of aspects of daily life, including food intake, exercise, and medication. People with diabetes can better manage their condition and gain valuable insights into their health by keeping track of these important factors. In order to effectively monitor and manage these aspects, we will examine the significance of tracking food intake, exercise, and medication for diabetes control and offer helpful hints.

FOLLOWING FOOD ADMISSION:

Segment Sizes:

In order to control blood sugar levels, it is essential to monitor portion sizes. Food can be measured or weighed to help people keep track of their carbohydrate intake, which has a big effect on blood sugar levels. The process can be made easier by utilizing food scales, measuring cups, or smartphone apps designed for portion control.

Sugar Counting:

Counting carbohydrates is a common diabetes management strategy. Monitoring starch admission permits people to match their insulin or medicine portions likewise. To determine the amount of carbohydrates in various foods, consult nutrition databases, food labels, or smartphone apps.

Glycemic List:

Foods' glycemic index (GI) can be used to learn more about how they affect blood sugar levels. Blood sugar levels are increased more quickly by foods with a high GI than by foods with a low GI. In order to effectively manage blood sugar levels, people can make better choices by tracking the GI of the foods they consume.

Feast Timing:

For diabetes control, it's important to eat at regular times. Individuals can identify patterns in blood sugar fluctuations and make necessary adjustments by tracking when they eat and snack.

EXERCISE IN TRACKING:

Time And Strenuousness: To learn how physical activity affects blood sugar levels, keep an eye on how much and how long you exercise. Before, during, and after exercise, keep track of the types of exercise, duration, and any changes in blood sugar levels. For better blood sugar control, this information can help determine the ideal exercise routine and timing.

Reaction to Exercise: Following glucose levels during and after practice assists people with understanding how their body answers various exercises. It can reveal patterns, like exercise-induced hypoglycemia or hyperglycemia, and help you make changes to your medication or how much carbohydrate you eat to keep your blood sugar levels stable.

. Assortment of Exercises: Participating in various proactive tasks offers various medical advantages. Individuals can ensure that they incorporate aerobic, strength, and flexibility training into their routines by tracking various types of exercises. Overall fitness and improved diabetes management are both aided by this.

MEDICATION MONITORING:

Dosage And Timing:

In order to effectively manage diabetes, it is essential to adhere to medication schedules. Keeping track of when and how much they take their medications helps people stay organized and ensures that they take them as directed. Tools like pill organizers, medication tracking apps, and smartphone reminders can be useful.

Incidental Effects And Viability :

Checking any secondary effects or changes in side effects connected with drug is significant. Individuals should talk to their doctor or other healthcare provider if they notice any adverse effects or changes in how their blood sugar is controlled. In order to achieve optimal diabetes management, this information aids healthcare professionals in modifying medication regimens.

Glucose Levels in the Blood:

Consistently following glucose levels related to drug use gives experiences into the viability of the treatment plan. It helps people and healthcare providers figure out if they need to change their medications to get their blood sugar levels in the right range.

BENEFITS OF KEEPING TRACK:

Identifying Examples: Individuals can identify patterns and trends in the management of their diabetes by keeping track of their food intake, exercise, and medication. They might notice, for instance, that certain foods consistently cause spikes in blood sugar, or that certain exercises make blood sugar levels more stable. Perceiving these examples empowers people to in like manner go with informed decisions and designer their diabetes the board techniques.

APPLICATION OF TECHNOLOGY TO THE MANAGEMENT OF DIABETES

To achieve optimal blood sugar control, diabetes management necessitates regular monitoring and thoughtful decision-making. The way diabetics manage their condition has been transformed by technological advancements. Technology provides a variety of tools that can simplify diabetes management, improve self-care, and provide useful insights for better control, including blood glucose monitoring devices and mobile applications. In this article, we will investigate the different manners by which innovation can be used for diabetes the executives and its advantages.

SYSTEMS FOR CONTINUOUS GLUCOSE MONITORING (CGM):

Wearable Continuous Glucose Monitoring (CGM) systems provide real-time blood sugar levels information. These gadgets use sensors embedded under the skin to gauge glucose levels in the interstitial liquid. Continuous glucose monitors (CGMs) make it possible for individuals to monitor changes in blood sugar levels, identify patterns, and make educated decisions regarding the management of their diabetes. Some CGMs even come equipped with alarms that let users know when their blood sugar levels are too high or too low, making them safer and easier to use.

METERS FOR BLOOD GLUCOSE:

Blood glucose meters are minimized gadgets utilized for self-checking glucose levels. For analysis, they typically require a small blood sample to be applied to a test strip. Memory storage is a feature of modern blood glucose meters that enables users to keep track of and examine their blood sugar readings over time. A few meters might be associated with cell phone applications, making it more straightforward to record and dissect glucose information. People are able to make well-informed choices regarding their diet, medications, and lifestyle choices if they monitor their blood sugar levels on a regular basis.

PUMPS FOR INSULIN:

An insulin pump is a small device that continuously delivers insulin via a tiny catheter inserted under the skin. Because these pumps enable precise insulin dosing, they give patients more control over their insulin therapy. Additionally, bolus calculators, which allow users to calculate insulin doses based on their blood sugar levels and carbohydrate intake, are built into many insulin pumps. A closed-loop system that automatically adjusts insulin delivery based on real-time glucose readings can be created by integrating some pumps with CGM systems.

APPS FOR MOBILE DEVICES:

Apps, or mobile applications, have evolved into potent diabetes management tools. There are various diabetes the board applications accessible that deal highlights, for example, glucose following, carb counting, drug updates, and feast arranging. These apps frequently sync with other devices, such as CGM systems or blood glucose meters, facilitating seamless data integration. In addition, some apps enable users to share data with healthcare providers, offer personalized recommendations, and offer educational resources, all of which contribute to improved diabetes care collaboration and communication.

REMOTE MONITORING AND TELEMEDICINE:

Diabetes patients now have access to remote consultations with healthcare professionals through the growing field of telemedicine. Individuals can discuss diabetes management, review blood sugar data, and receive treatment plan guidance via video calls or online platforms. Healthcare professionals can quickly make adjustments to the treatment plan and access blood sugar readings, insulin pump data, or CGM data through remote monitoring systems.

COMPUTERIZED REASONING (MAN-MADE INTELLIGENCE) AND INFORMATION EXAMINATION:

Man-made consciousness (computer based intelligence) calculations and information examination methods can possibly change diabetes the executives. AI systems can provide personalized insights and predictive models to support decision-making by analyzing vast amounts of data. For instance, artificial intelligence calculations can investigate blood glucose designs, dietary propensities, active work, and prescription use to distinguish patterns, give proposals, and anticipate future glucose levels. People may be able to benefit from such systems by making proactive adjustments to their diabetes management and avoiding potential complications.

WEARABLE GADGETS AND WELLNESS TRACKERS:

For diabetes management, wearable devices like smartwatches and fitness trackers offer additional advantages. Physical activity, sleep patterns, heart rate, and even stress levels can all be tracked by these gadgets.

Celebrating milestones and remaining motivated Diabetes management necessitates consistent effort, dedication, and commitment. There are numerous achievements and milestones to be recognized as one works toward diabetes control. Diabetes patients can maintain a positive outlook, persist in their efforts, and continue to place a high priority on their health and well-being by recognizing these milestones and remaining motivated. In this article, we'll talk about how important it is to celebrate milestones and how to keep yourself motivated to control your diabetes.

RECOGNIZING PROGRESS:

Recognizing and appreciating each step forward in diabetes management is important. This includes achieving the desired levels of blood sugar, losing weight, successfully incorporating exercise into a routine, and following a medication schedule. People can boost their self-confidence and reinforce positive behaviors by recognizing these accomplishments.

REALISTIC OBJECTIVES:

To stay motivated, it's important to set goals that are attainable. Breaking down long-term objectives into smaller, more manageable milestones can give you a sense of accomplishment along the way. For instance, rather than aiming to lose a lot of weight, people can set a goal to lose a certain number of pounds in a certain amount of time. By recognizing these smaller victories, momentum and motivation for continued progress are created.

INCENTIVES AND REWARDS:

A powerful motivator is rewarding oneself for achieving milestones. Set up a system of rewards that matches your preferences and interests. Prizes can go from basic deals with like a most loved dinner or a loosening up spa day to buying another wellness contraption or booking an end of the week escape. The most important thing is to pick rewards that make you happy and make you want to work harder at controlling your diabetes.

SHARE ACCOMPLISHMENTS:

Imparting accomplishments to friends and family, companions, or a diabetes support local area can produce a feeling of satisfaction and inspiration. Social help assumes a vital part in diabetes the board, and praising achievements together cultivates a feeling of local area and support. To connect with others on a similar journey, think about sharing accomplishments on social media, joining support groups, or attending local diabetes events.

MONITORING CHANGES:

A good way to stay motivated and monitor diabetes control is to track progress. Use different apparatuses, for example, versatile applications, diaries, or calculation sheets to record glucose levels, medicine adherence, work-out schedules, and dietary propensities. A visual representation of progress and a spotlight on areas in need of improvement are provided by regularly reviewing these records. It can be extremely motivating to witness tangible evidence of positive changes.

KNOWLEDGE AND TRAINING:

Motivation can be boosted by continuously expanding one's knowledge of diabetes and how to manage it. To keep up with the most recent research, treatment options, and self-care practices, take diabetes education classes, workshops, or seminars. People who are aware of how lifestyle choices, medications, and exercise affect blood sugar control are better able to make educated choices and remain motivated to manage their diabetes.

SEEK ADVICE FROM A PROFESSIONAL:

Engaging in conversation with healthcare professionals like endocrinologists, diabetes educators, or dietitians can be very helpful for getting advice and support. Monitoring progress, making adjustments to treatment plans, and receiving expert advice tailored to each patient's needs are all made possible by regular checkups. These communications act as tokens of the significance of progressing diabetes control and can reignite inspiration to keep rolling out sure improvements.

EMBRACE A POSITIVE OUTLOOK:

For long-term diabetes management, it is essential to maintain a positive outlook. Recognize the possibility of failure, but view them as opportunities for growth rather than setbacks. Concentrate on the progress that has been made and the possibility of further progress. Practice positive self-talk, encircle yourself with steady people, and take part in exercises that advance mental prosperity, like care reflection or journaling.

PARTICIPATE IN FUN ACTIVITIES:

For overall well-being and motivation, engaging in enjoyable activities unrelated to diabetes management is essential. Spend time on pastimes, interests, and activities that make you happy and help you unwind.

All in all, while diabetes is a persistent condition that ordinarily requires continuous clinical administration, there are different procedures people can embrace to help their diabetes the executives and in general wellbeing. The procedures examined in this article center around making way of life changes that can decidedly affect glucose control, insulin awareness, and generally prosperity.

A reasonable eating regimen that stresses entire food varieties, segment control, and restricting handled food varieties and sweet refreshments is significant. Improved insulin sensitivity and improved blood sugar management are both benefits of regular aerobic and strength training exercise. If you are overweight, working toward weight loss or maintaining a healthy weight can significantly improve your diabetes control.

In conclusion, for overall health and blood sugar management, stress management techniques like meditation, deep breathing exercises, engaging in enjoyable activities, and prioritizing quality sleep are essential. Normal observing of glucose levels, adherence to recommended meds, and looking for help from medical care experts and encouraging groups of people likewise assume a fundamental part in diabetes the board.

It is essential to keep in mind that these methods are meant to complement rather than replace medical treatment. Diabetes patients must collaborate closely with their healthcare team, which includes endocrinologists, primary care physicians, and diabetes educators, to develop an individual management plan that takes into account their particular requirements and objectives.

By embracing these methods and making feasible way of life changes, people can play a functioning job in their diabetes the board, further develop glucose control, and improve their general personal satisfaction. Although there is no cure for diabetes, ongoing self-care, medical treatment, and healthy lifestyle choices can significantly influence its management.

It's important to remember that every person's diabetes experience is different, and what works for one person might not work for another. It is absolutely necessary to pay attention to your body, monitor your progress, and adjust as necessary. With devotion, tirelessness, and a promise to a solid way of life, people can really deal with their diabetes and lead satisfying, dynamic lives.

Keep in mind, assuming you have diabetes, talk with your medical services group for customized exhortation and direction. They can give you the most accurate information and help you get the best care for your diabetes. You can effectively manage diabetes while living a full life by taking charge of your health and making wise choices.

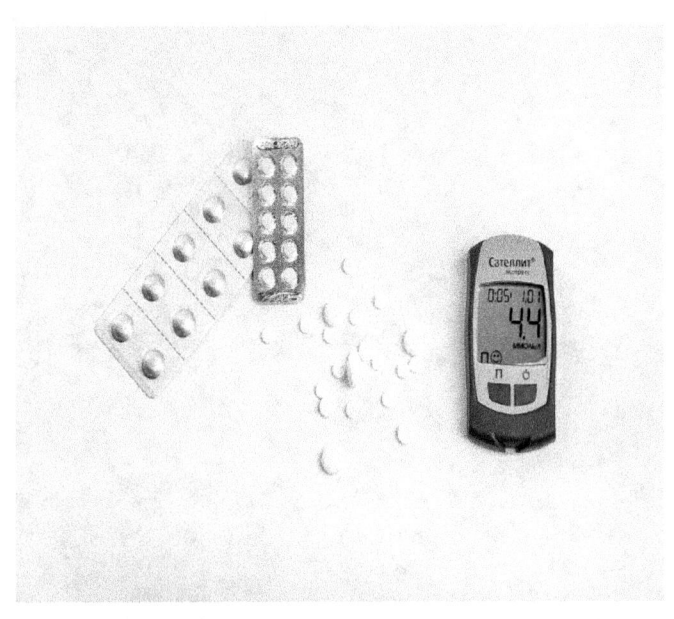